NEW DIRECTIONS FOR

MW01168613

H. Richard Lamb, *University of Southern California*
EDITOR-IN-CHIEF

Families Coping with Mental Illness: The Cultural Context

Harriet P. Lefley
University of Miami School of Medicine

EDITOR

Number 77, Spring 1998

JOSSEY-BASS PUBLISHERS
San Francisco

FAMILIES COPING WITH MENTAL ILLNESS: THE CULTURAL CONTEXT
Harriet P. Lefley (ed.)
New Directions for Mental Health Services, no. 77
H. Richard Lamb, Editor-in-Chief

Microfilm copies of issues and articles are available in 16mm and 35mm, as well as microfiche in 105mm, through University Microfilms Inc., 300 North Zeeb Road, Ann Arbor, Michigan 48106-1346.

ISSN 0193-9416   ISBN 0-7879-1426-6

NEW DIRECTIONS FOR MENTAL HEALTH SERVICES is part of The Jossey-Bass Psychology Series and is published quarterly by Jossey-Bass Inc., Publishers, 350 Sansome Street, San Francisco, California 94104–1342.

SUBSCRIPTIONS cost $63.00 for individuals and $105.00 for institutions, agencies, and libraries.

EDITORIAL CORRESPONDENCE should be sent to the Editor-in-Chief, H. Richard Lamb, University of Southern California, Department of Psychiatry, Graduate Hall, 1937 Hospital Place, Los Angeles, California 90033–1071.

Cover photograph by Wernher Krutein/PHOTOVAULT © 1990.

Jossey-Bass Web address: www.josseybass.com

Printed in the United States of America on acid-free recycled paper containing 100 percent recovered waste paper, of which at least 20 percent is postconsumer waste.

CONTENTS

EDITOR'S NOTES

This issue of *New Directions for Mental Health Services* offers both a longitudinal and a cross-sectional perspective on the involvement of families in the treatment of adults with severe and persistent psychiatric disorders. Mental illness is experienced, both by patients and by their families, in a historical and cultural context that varies across time, geography, personal space, and the life cycle of the illness. This sourcebook views culture in the broadest sense, as a set of shared beliefs, values, behavioral norms, and practices that characterize a particular group of people who share a common identity and the symbolic meanings of a common language. Although the definition of culture has typically been restricted to ethnicity, social scientists recognize many subcultures based on social roles. These include professions whose members have a shared belief system, a common symbolic idiom, and consensually standardized practices. In the understanding and treatment of major mental illness, there have been profound changes in the cultures of mental health professionals and the clinical systems in which they serve. Changing beliefs and practices with respect to family roles, and families' increasing involvement in knowledge acquisition, treatment planning, self-help programs, and patient advocacy are part of a new knowledge base and new views of the appropriate alliance for patient care. This is the sociocultural context—a product of empirical research, changing service needs, increased consumer influence, and altered role relationships.

Embedded in the context of changing practices is the question of ethnic differences, both within and across nations. There is now a substantial literature on ethnocultural variation in the definitions, manifestations, social perceptions, treatment, and prognoses of mental illness. As with all social science applications, we do not know how constant these descriptions are. It is unclear to what extent different ethnocultural perceptions might persist in a global village with instant access to information, collaborative research, shared training models, and the fluid epistemology of a planet undergoing rapid industrialization. The world is rapidly changing, and new knowledge brings adaptations of former convictions. In the Western world we see ongoing revision of older theories and treatments of the major psychiatric disorders and massive adjustments in service delivery systems as a result of managed care. All of these factors have an impact on the professional culture of mental health care providers and on the parameters of therapeutic intervention.

Accordingly, this sourcebook discusses cultural beliefs and practices in reference to the changing context of mental health theory and treatment, and also with respect to ethnic diversity, as culture is commonly interpreted. In the sociocultural context, the past twenty years have seen enormous changes in knowledge about the major psychiatric disorders and the family's role. The field has in general gone from excluding families to welcoming them into the treatment process, from interventions based on presumptive family psychopathology to education and support services to relieve the family's burden. Families' roles in political advocacy have generated new self-help models, including interventions that focus on family well-being rather than the family as an adjunct to patient care.

But the descriptions in this sourcebook are also sensitive to the ethnocultural context, to research and interventions with different ethnic minority groups. For this reason there are specific contributions relevant to work with families of persons with severe mental illness who are African American, American Indian, Asian (Indochinese), and Hispanic as well as white American. We can see from these contributions that caregivers in these groups may differ in defining and evaluating their loved one's disability and how it should be treated. There are differences in the parameters of social support, in caregiving obligations, and in perceptions of family burden. These findings have clinical relevance as well as implications for social policy. It is hoped that the two broad foci, the sociocultural and ethnocultural perspectives, will suggest new ways of conceptualizing the family's role and that this understanding will enrich professional-family relationships in a collaborative therapeutic enterprise.

Harriet P. Lefley
Editor

HARRIET P. LEFLEY is professor of psychiatry and behavioral sciences, University of Miami School of Medicine.

PART ONE

The Sociocultural Context of Family Interventions

This chapter provides an overview of interventions for relatives of severely mentally ill individuals. The author discusses the design and use of these interventions in the context of the cultural characteristics of families and providers, as well as the culture of the interventions themselves.

The Cultural Context of Interventions for Family Members with a Seriously Mentally Ill Relative

Phyllis Solomon

A society's beliefs about major psychiatric illness determine how families with an adult relative with a severe mental illness are treated. Cultural belief systems surrounding mental illness influence whether families are informed about the illness, its course, and treatment; whether they are included in the treatment process; and whether providers make any special effort to ease their stress and responsibilities in caring for their relative and managing the illness. This chapter discusses the history and cultural context of the mental health system's beliefs regarding families with a mentally ill relative and the implications of the system's culture for family interventions. It also provides a programmatic definition of family interventions and discusses the implications for the design and use of family interventions of the cultural context of providers, families, and intervention processes and structures. The chapter concludes with an examination of the impact of family interventions on cultural beliefs about adults with severe mental illness and their families, both in the wider society and in the mental health system in particular.

Historical Context of Family Interventions

In the era of asylums families were considered passive contributors to the onset of mental illness for not having protected their relative from societal disorganization, which was believed to be the principal causal agent (Terkelsen, 1990). Separation from the family was only one element in the process of shielding the patient from the confusion and pressures of the larger society

(Terkelsen, 1990). Subsequently, families, particularly parents, were viewed as the causal agents of these disorders. Based on these psychodynamic theories, separation of the ill relative from his or her family persisted, as it was considered essential to helping the patient resolve "issues of parental pathogenesis" (Lefley, 1996, p. 16). As a result of these explanations, families were not only ignored and left uninformed about their relative's diagnosis and treatment but also were blamed for the illness.

Over time there was a reversal in thinking from complete isolation of the patient from the family as a means of treating the patient to a need to modify the dynamics of the family's interactions. From this conceptualization emerged the need for family therapy to treat the dysfunctional family (Lefley, 1996; Terkelsen, 1990). Families were then put in the position of being confronted with their responsibility for their relative's illness. Psychodynamic and family systems theories about the etiology of major psychiatric illnesses are evident in mental health settings even today (Terkelsen, 1990).

Despite the popularity of these psychogenic theories as explanations for the causes of major psychiatric disorders, their significance waned due to a lack of supporting evidence. Family therapies based on these conceptualizations did not demonstrate clinical benefits (Mueser and Glynn, forthcoming). Subsequently, there was a shift from belief in a single etiological cause to belief in a combination of biological and environmental factors that result in the onset and course of psychiatric disorders (Coursey, Alford, and Safarjan, 1997; Lehman, Thompson, Dixon, and Scott, 1995). These biopsychosocial explanatory models of vulnerability or stress diathesis inspired comprehensive treatment programs consisting of medication for patients and psychosocial treatment for their families.

The development of psychosocial interventions for families of adults with severe mental illness was stimulated by research that found that recently released patients who returned to families who were highly critical, overinvolved, and hostile or labeled as high in expressed emotion (EE) were more likely to relapse than those who returned to low-EE families (Mueser and Glynn, forthcoming; Vaughn and Leff, 1976; Brown, Birley, and Wing, 1972). These findings precipitated a host of investigations of randomized controlled trials of family interventions to change the family environment and reduce patient relapse (Dixon and Lehman, 1995; Lam, 1991; Strachan, 1986; Hogarty, Anderson, and Reiss, 1987). There is much controversy surrounding this research, however, as it continues to blame families, and the direction of causality of high EE is unclear (Hatfield, Spaniol, and Zipple, 1987; Mintz, Liberman, Miklowitz, and Mintz, 1987).

In an independent effort, families who were dissatisfied with the treatment provided to their relative, the lack of communication between themselves and their family member's mental health care providers, and provider attitudes toward families came together in various locales across the country to form support and advocacy groups (Shetler, 1986). The exponential growth in these groups was undoubtedly stimulated by deinstitutionalization, which left the care of ill relatives largely up to their families. The social stigma associated with mental illness resulted in isolation of families, who feared the repercussions of disclosing their relative's illness to others. These families met to share experiences and find support. Individuals from these grassroots support groups met in 1979 in Madison, Wisconsin, to form a national coalition of these independent groups, the National Alliance for the Mentally Ill (NAMI) (Shetler, 1986). NAMI not only advocates for legislative changes but also has been the impetus for an enormous expansion of local support groups.

Defining Family Interventions

The emergence of family interventions reflects a shift from viewing families as the cause of mental illness to viewing them as a resource and a source of support for their ill relative (Marsh and Johnson, 1997). To some extent this shift was necessitated by the deinstitutionalization movement, which as noted previously left families the de facto caregivers for their ill relatives, a role for which they had no training or knowledge and that often brought enormous stress and burdens. A family intervention in such cases can be defined as any strategy or program, clinical or nonclinical, designed to help and empower these families to cope with these devastating disorders through such means as the provision of support, education, and skill training. Family interventions may be provided by professionals or nonprofessionals, including family members themselves. Diverse interventions meet this definition, including psychoeducation, family education, family consultation, family support and advocacy groups, and other forms of assistance to families, including marital and family therapy and respite care. Although only psychoeducation has been extensively researched, all of these interventions are generally perceived as helpful by family members, as they serve different functions.

Types of Family Interventions

There is a diverse array of family interventions that are clinical as well as nonclinical. The following discussion provides an overview of these interventions.

Psychoeducation. Psychoeducation models are typically a component of a comprehensive treatment program for the ill relative (Solomon, 1996). Most interventions draw on social learning, behavioral, and cognitive theory. If relevant, they may focus on reduction of high EE, although interventions are needed by low-EE families as well. All psychoeducational models include "education about the illness, support for families, problem-solving strategies, and illness management techniques" (Lefley, 1996, p. 132). For some interventions the ill relative is present; others include separate sessions for the ill family member. All are designed, delivered, and evaluated by professionals (sometimes a team of professionals). Many are delivered in clinical settings, but some are delivered in the family's home. These interventions usually require a relatively long-term commitment on the part of the family, anywhere from nine months to two years or more. They are often initiated at a crisis point for the family, such as during hospitalization or upon discharge. The educational component may be an initial step toward entering traditional family therapy. For the most part these interventions have been research efforts. In most mental health systems they have not become a part of routine treatment, although their efficacy has been demonstrated (Dixon and Lehman, 1995).

Family Consultation (Supportive Family Counseling). Family consultation is often provided by a professional but sometimes by a trained family member. The consultant offers expert advice and information either to an individual family member or to the whole family unit (Bernheim, 1982; Bernheim and Lehman, 1985; Kanter, 1985). This is a flexible and collaborative approach to working with families (Marsh and Johnson, 1997). As adapted by the Training and Education Center (TEC) Network of Philadelphia, this intervention has three phases. In the first phase, of feeling or connecting, the consultant takes a brief history of the relative's illness, offers empathy and support, acknowledges family strengths, addresses issues of guilt and blame, and assesses the family's need for education and skill development. In the next, or focusing, phase, the consultant develops an agenda for the family's educational program, clarifies its problems, and creates a prioritized list of objectives. In the final, or finding, phase, the consultant helps the family develop strategies for meeting the agreed-upon objectives. Besides helping family members develop new skills, the consultant might also evaluate their use of those skills in relating to the ill relative, inform them about appropriate community resources, and occasionally accompany them to meetings with service agencies (Mannion, Meisel, Draine, and Solomon, forthcoming). TEC provides some of these services by phone, and recently it adapted this model to a group format (Mannion, Meisel, Draine, and Solomon, forthcoming). The structure and process of TEC's group-format intervention is similar to the multifamily approach, except that the ill family member is not included in the TEC model (McFarlane and others, 1995).

Family Education. Family education is a nonclinical intervention that has a strengths approach as its theoretical base, with stress reduction, improved coping, and adaptation as its targeted outcomes. In contrast to psychoeducation, which was designed to meet the needs of the ill relative, family education was developed primarily to meet the needs of families. These programs come from an adult learning and health promotion orientation. Family education does not presume any family dysfunction, as does the more medical emphasis of some psychoeducational models. Goals of this intervention are to increase the family's knowledge of the disorder, increase their coping skills, alleviate their burden and stress, and improve quality of life for them and their ill relative (Hatfield, 1994; Solomon, 1996). Family education is generally implemented in a group format, with didactic lectures the primary format, perhaps supplemented with audio or visual aids. Frequently these interventions also include experiential elements, offering participants the opportunity to practice the skills being taught. They are usually short-term interventions, consisting of anywhere from a couple of hours in a single day to multiple two- or three-hour sessions over a ten- or twelve-week period. These interventions have been developed and delivered by professionals, by family members, and by a combination of the two. Generally the ill relative is not a participant, so families can be comfortable in discussing their concerns. The group format offers support, empathy, and a chance to share experiences. Many such interventions arise from freestanding grassroots efforts; others are part of mental health programs. The research on these programs is very limited, but they show promise in terms of achieving their goals (Solomon, 1996; Solomon, Draine, Mannion, and Meisel, 1996, 1997). The most noted family education program, currently offered in numerous communities nationwide, is NAMI's Family-to-Family program (formerly called the Journey of Hope; see Chapter Three).

Family Support and Advocacy Groups. Family support groups are an essential nonclinical intervention for families of adults with severe mental illness (Lefley, 1996). They provide support, information, understanding, and opportunities to pursue advocacy (Marsh and Johnson, 1997). Member-facilitated group sessions offer contact with others who have shared similar experiences. Members share resources, information, coping strategies, and ideas for managing their ill relative (Lefley, 1996). Frequently these groups sponsor lectures and educational programs. Families often want more from these groups than simply a forum for sharing their grief and pain. They want to move toward action. Specifically, members want "to eradicate mental illness, to change the system, to provide needed services, to fight stigma, to obtain a better quality of life for their loved ones" (Lefley, 1996, p. 141). Advocacy gives purpose and meaning to the lives of these families and becomes a therapeutic tool for them. These families therefore advocate for a variety of policy and legislative changes at both the local and national levels.

Other Interventions. There are also other, more specialized interventions, such as one for children of parents with serious affective disorders (Lefley, 1996). There are financial planning programs for parents wondering how to provide for the future of an ill adult child, and respite care, which offers families relief from the stresses of caregiving. In some instances there may be a need to develop interventions in response to specific issues. For example, in certain situations families resort to the use of restraining orders (Solomon, Draine, and Delaney, 1995); a mediation intervention may be effective in such cases to prevent the need for future restraining orders.

The family interventions discussed here are generally educational and supportive, serving the family's needs for information, skill acquisition, and emotional support. When these services are not sufficient, individual, family, and marital therapy are also available (Marsh and Johnson, 1997). Although these types of interventions might not help a family relate to their ill relative, they can help family members deal with personal problems resulting from or exacerbated by having a relative with severe mental illness (Lefley, 1996; Marsh and Johnson, 1997).

In addition, family interventions can be incorporated into other services, such as case management (Solomon, Draine, Mannion, and Meisel, 1997). For example, multifamily group therapy has been integrated into an assertive community treatment (ACT) case management program, Family-Aided Assertive Community Treatment (FACT); integrating a crisis family intervention into an ACT program is another alternative (McFarlane and others, 1996). McFarlane and his colleagues note that inclusion of the family in the treatment process differed from the orientation of the original program model, which emphasized "constructive separation" of the client from the family. This separation was based on the premise that crisis resolution would be hindered if the ill relative interacted with his or her family (1996).

The Impact of Family Culture

Ethnicity is a major determinant of people's belief systems. It influences families' beliefs about what causes mental illness and their attitudes toward mental health care providers. A family's ethnicity also has an impact on which interventions are likely to resolve their problems related to a family member's disorder. Furthermore, the definition of what constitutes a family differs by cultural groups (McGoldrick, 1982), as do the roles different family members assume within the family context. These factors in turn affect families' behaviors during mental health interventions and the types of interventions they are willing to pursue. Certain ethnic groups, particularly African Americans and other minority groups, have not participated in family interventions to any great extent. This has been the situation with clinical interventions, such as psychoeducation, as well as nonclinical ones, such as family education and support groups. This has also been the situation in research on these interventions and other related issues, such as burden and caregiving relief. As a consequence, the effectiveness of these interventions for minority groups is unclear.

For family interventions to be attractive to the diverse array of families with a relative with severe mental illness, they must be sensitive to cultural variations. Deciding whether interventions should be designed by families, by professionals, or jointly requires a consideration of a variety of family cultures, as cultural issues influence the "accessibility and acceptability" of mental health services (Guarnaccia and Parra, 1996). In addition, some approaches may not be sufficient for certain groups. For example, Lefley (1990) indicates that structured family therapy, which helps to restore traditional family relationships, may be more beneficial than psychoeducation for immigrant groups in which role changes are eroding the established family structure. Jordan, Lewellen, and Vandiver (1995) delineate particular considerations and recommendations for family education programs for Laotian, African American, and Mexican American families.

One factor of importance to be considered in the design of such programs is the cultural definition of a family. For example, in some cultures the family may go beyond the nuclear family to the extended family. It may also be important for members of some cultural groups to include folk healers, priests, and other nonblood members, such as godparents, in family interventions (Jordan, Lewellen, and Vandiver, 1995). Sharing problems with strangers may be inherently antithetical to some groups' values. In these situations a family consultation model may be more appropriate than a group approach. Cultural sensitivity on the part of the provider is crucial in making appropriate referrals, modifying existing interventions, and developing new ones. Providers may be inaccurate in assuming a family needs a particular intervention. The family may need the information or support a particular intervention can provide, but this does not necessarily mean they need that intervention, as another may be culturally more suitable.

Also, families from some cultures may not feel a need for emotional support from strangers, since they have an extended support system consisting of friends and their church. Research by Pickett, Vraniak, Cook, and Cohler (1993) found that black families accommodate and adjust to an ill child more readily than white families. The explanation these investigators put forth was that blacks may not hold "normative-development expectations regarding age-appropriate behavior" to the same extent as white families (p. 465). Some cultures do not find the term *mental illness* acceptable, and other cultures may find it disrespectful to set limits on older family members. Consequently, different terminology and program structures may be necessary for particular cultural groups (Lundwall, 1996). It remains an open question whether effective groups need to be culturally homogenous (Shankar, 1994); however, maintaining group homogeneity may be essential to attract families from a particular culture and ensure their comfort with the process.

For the most part all of these interventions, both the clinical and the nonclinical ones, are designed for parents with an adult child with severe mental illness (mainly schizophrenia). Since people with psychiatric illness now spend the majority of their time in the community and are having children of their own, these interventions require modifications. Family members with different relationships to the mentally ill individual have different role interactions and responsibilities and thus need different information and support. Mannion, Mueser, and Solomon (1994) point out the importance of specifically designing programs for spouses of someone with a severe mental illness. Frequently when spouses do attend a local NAMI meeting they do not stay long enough to get involved or to realize that other spouses do occasionally show up (Mannion, Mueser, and Solomon, 1994; Mannion, 1996). The needs of siblings of mentally ill individuals have often been overlooked in educational and support interventions (Lundwall, 1996). Likewise, adult children of mentally ill individuals have been neglected by family education efforts, and interventions for younger children require still more modification.

The Impact of Professional Culture

Clinicians' attitudes toward families are a product of their clinical training (Lefley, 1990). Due to a variety of factors, including recent research, negative views regarding the role families play in the etiology and management of their relatives' illness have changed; nevertheless, some mental health professionals continue to reject and ignore families (Lefley, 1988, 1996). This results from the fact that some of those who were trained during an earlier time continue to practice and teach without updating themselves on current research. Furthermore, training programs are a reflection of the values, theories, and research interests of their institutional faculty and administrations (Lefley, 1990). One family therapist who works effectively with families of adults with severe mental illness frequently comments that she is a "recovering" family therapist; in other words, she is recovering from her training in the area of working with families of persons with a severe mental illness. Inevitably the professional and personal values of practitioners, including their own cultural socialization, influence the design of any program they develop. Similarly, these same values also play a role in the information they provide about these interventions and in which patients they refer to them. For example, practitioners can use confidentiality issues to justify not working with families, rather than attempting to resolve this professional conflict (see Marsh and Johnson, 1997, for ways to resolve potential confidentiality problems in working with families). There are a number of opportunities for practitioners to update themselves on recent developments in family interventions and family research, should their values move them in this direction.

Cultural Aspects of the Design and Use of Interventions

Interventions, too, have cultures, insofar as the participants share attitudes, values, goals, and practices. For individual interventions the practitioner's and family members' engagement and their commitment to forming an alliance affect the rates of retention and the benefits of the intervention to the family. The degree of alliance is contingent on shared beliefs and goals between the family and the practitioner. In addition, whether the intervention is delivered in the home, a clinic, or another setting, as well as the auspices under which it is offered, affect the culture of the intervention and thus its attractiveness to families and rate of retention. The availability and accessibility of the intervention is also crucial to its attractiveness to families. For some families home-delivered or over-the-phone interventions are far more attractive and comfortable. Budd and Hughes (1997) found that one of the most helpful aspects of family interventions was families' knowing that they could contact the practitioner for help and advice should problems or difficulties arise.

The factors that influence group interventions' cultures are somewhat more complicated. Factors such as group size, participation of the ill relative, setting, administrative auspices, degree of homogeneity of the membership, and whether the group is led by a professional or by a family member affect the intervention's attractiveness and the retention of family members. Hatfield (1997) noted that NAMI members are raising questions with regard to which characteristics are appropriate for sorting participants of support groups. Participants of support groups are frequently diverse with regard to "age of care-giver and ill relative, length of illness, caregiver relationship to ill member, diagnoses, ethnicity, and other characteristics" (p. 259). Leaders feel that groups should be more homogeneous for participants to optimally benefit, but as of yet there has been no research regarding which group member charac-teristics need to be the same. These issues are relevant not only for support groups but also for educational and therapy groups.

The length of time a group has been in existence and the degree of turnover in the group also affect the intervention's culture. Families are initially attracted to support groups to meet their needs for information and support, but as these needs are met, members tend to move toward a desire for advo-cacy. When families with a recently diagnosed relative attend a local support group that focuses on advocacy, they frequently do not return after their ini-tial meeting (Citron, Solomon, and Draine, forthcoming). Some groups now recognize this evolutionary change toward advocacy in intervention cultures and designate a particular member to spend time with new attendees. This is a potential solution to the problem of retaining new members, as it offers new participants an opportunity to develop a relationship with the group by hav-ing someone to listen to their concerns and share experiences with.

The Feedback Loop: The Impact of Family Interventions on Stigma and Views About Families

As family interventions for adults with severe mental illness have exponentially increased, these interventions have had an impact on society's view of adults with severe mental illness and their families. For example, the advocacy efforts of NAMI and its local affiliates, directed at educating the public in general and federal and state legislators in particular, have improved people's understand-ing of mental illness as a brain disease and resulted in increased empathy for families. Similarly, NAMI's antistigma campaign has made the public more aware of some of the myths and inaccuracies surrounding mental illness that have been perpetuated by the media.

These interventions also offer families increased understanding of their ill relative's disorders and greater confidence in their ability to assertively voice their and their relative's needs to providers in the mental health system. Fam-ilies that are well-informed, articulate, and willing to communicate essential information regarding their relative's symptoms and behaviors contribute much to changing provider attitudes. Consequently, interventions that educate fam-ilies have the potential to improve the mental health system, both for individ-uals with mental illness and for their families. With a receptive attitude toward families, providers can learn much from collaborating with them, in terms of developing the most beneficial interventions for patients and in terms of plan-ning services and strategies for working with family members. Even without highly structured interventions for families, family-provider collaboration serves the best interests of everyone.

For too long the mental health system has either ignored or blamed the family. Frequently when family members *are* considered it is only in the context of what they can provide their ill relative, whether it be housing or financial or emotional support. If family members are assessed as needing help themselves, they are typically referred to existing services or treatments, such as family or marital therapy, rather than offered interventions responsive to their specific needs and desires.

This chapter has hopefully achieved its purpose of spreading the message that family interventions are quite varied and consequently have value for a wide array of families. Furthermore, most families can benefit from education, support, and training in coping and management strategies. However, for the greatest number of families to benefit from such interventions, the cultural context of the families and of the interventions themselves need to be taken into consideration, both in the design and development of the interventions and in referral practices. Providers cannot continue to adopt a procrustean approach to meeting the needs of families with a relative with severe mental illness. There is a plethora of helpful family interventions that can be adapted from the existing array of models. The one-size-fits-all approach will not best serve the diversity of families affected by a relative with a severe psychiatric disorder.

References

Bernheim, K. F. "Supportive Family Counseling." *Schizophrenia Bulletin,* 1982, *8,* 634–640.

Bernheim, K. F., and Lehman, A. *Working with Families of the Mentally Ill.* New York: Norton, 1985.

Brown, G., Birley, J., and Wing, J. "Influence of Psychiatric Illness." *British Journal of Psychiatry,* 1972, *121,* 241–258.

Budd, R., and Hughes, I. "What Do Relatives of People with Schizophrenia Find Helpful About Family Intervention?" *Schizophrenia Bulletin,* 1997, *23,* 341–347.

Citron, M., Solomon, P., and Draine, J. "Self-Help Groups for Families of Persons with Mental Illness: Perceived Benefits of Helpfulness." *Community Mental Health Journal,* forthcoming.

Coursey, R., Alford, J., and Safarjan, B. "Significant Advances in Understanding and Treating Serious Mental Illness." *Professional Psychology: Research and Practice,* 1997, *28,* 205–216.

Dixon, L., and Lehman, A. "Family Interventions for Schizophrenia." *Schizophrenia Bulletin,* 1995, *21,* 631–643.

Guarnaccia, P., and Parra, P. "Ethnicity, Social Status, and Families' Experiences of Caring for a Mentally Ill Family Member." *Community Mental Health Journal,* 1996, *32,* 243–260.

Hatfield, A. B. "Family Education: Theory and Practice." In A. B. Hatfield (ed.), *Family Interventions in Mental Illness.* New Directions for Mental Health Services, no. 62. San Francisco: Jossey-Bass, 1994.

Hatfield, A. B. "Families of Adults with Severe Mental Illness: New Directions for Research." *American Journal of Orthopsychiatry,* 1997, *67,* 254–260.

Hatfield, A. B., Spaniol, L., and Zipple, A. "Expressed Emotion: A Family Perspective." *Schizophrenia Bulletin,* 1987, *13,* 221–226.

Hogarty, G., Anderson, C., and Reiss, D. "Family Psychoeducation, Social Skills Training, and Medication in Schizophrenia: The Long and Short of It." *Psychopharmacology Bulletin,* 1987, *23,* 12–13.

Jordan, C., Lewellen, A., and Vandiver, V. "Psychoeducation for Minority Families: A Social Work Perspective." *International Journal of Mental Health,* 1995, 23 (4), 27–43.

Kanter, J. "Consulting with Families of the Chronic Mentally Ill." In J. Kanter (ed.), *Clinical Issues in Treating the Chronic Mentally Ill.* New Directions for Mental Health Services, no. 27. San Francisco: Jossey-Bass, 1985.

Lam, D. "Psychosocial Family Interventions in Schizophrenia: A Review of Empirical Studies." *Psychological Medicine,* 1991, 21, 423–441.

Lefley, H. "Training Professionals to Work with Families of Chronic Patients." *Community Mental Health Journal,* 1988, 24, 338–357.

Lefley, H. "Cultural Issues in Training Psychiatric Residents to Work with Families of the Long-Term Mentally Ill." In E. Sorel (ed.), *Family, Culture and Psychobiology.* New York: Legas, 1990.

Lefley, H. *Family Caregiving in Mental Illness.* Thousand Oaks, Calif.: Sage, 1996.

Lehman, A., Thompson, J., Dixon, L., and Scott, J. "Schizophrenia: Treatment Outcomes Research." *Schizophrenia Bulletin,* 1995, 21, 561–566.

Lundwall, R. "How Psychoeducation Support Groups Can Provide Multidiscipline Services to Families of People with Mental Illness." *Psychiatric Rehabilitation Journal,* 1996, 20, 64–71.

Mannion, E. "Resilience and Burden in Spouses of People with Mental Illness." *Psychiatric Rehabilitation Journal,* 1996, 20, 13–23.

Mannion, E., Meisel, M., Draine, J., and Solomon, P. "Applying Research on Family Education About Mental Illness to Development of a Relative's Group Consultation Model." *Community Mental Health Journal,* forthcoming.

Mannion, E., Mueser, K., and Solomon, P. "Designing Psychoeducational Services for Spouses of Persons with Serious Mental Illness." *Community Mental Health Journal,* 1994, 30, 177–190.

Marsh, D., and Johnson, D. "The Family Experience of Mental Illness: Implications for Interventions." *Professional Psychology: Research and Practice,* 1997, 28, 229–237.

McFarlane, W., and others. "Psychoeducational Multiple Family Groups: Four-Year Relapse Outcome in Schizophrenia." *Family Process,* 1995, 34, 127–144.

McFarlane, W., and others. "A Comparison of Two Levels of Family-Aided Assertive Community Treatment." *Psychiatric Services,* 1996, 47, 744–750.

McGoldrick, M. "Ethnicity and Family Therapy: An Overview." In M. McGoldrick, J. Pearce, and J. Giordano (eds.), *Ethnicity and Family Therapy.* New York: Guilford Press, 1982.

Mintz, L., Liberman, R., Miklowitz, D., and Mintz, J. "Expressed Emotion: A Call for Partnership Among Relatives, Patients, and Professionals." *Schizophrenia Bulletin,* 1987, 13, 227–235.

Mueser, K., and Glynn, S. "Family Intervention for Schizophrenia." In K. S. Dobson and K. D. Craig (eds.), *Best Practice: Developing and Promoting Empirically Validated Interventions.* Thousand Oaks, Calif.: Sage, forthcoming.

Pickett, S., Vraniak, D., Cook, J., and Cohler, B. "Strength in Adversity: Blacks Bear Burden Better Than Whites." *Professional Psychology: Research and Practice,* 1993, 24, 460–467.

Shankar, R. "Interventions with Families of People with Schizophrenia in India." In A. B. Hatfield (ed.), *Family Interventions in Mental Illness.* New Directions for Mental Health Services, no. 62. San Francisco: Jossey-Bass, 1994.

Shetler, H. *A History of the National Alliance for the Mentally Ill.* Arlington, Va.: National Alliance for the Mentally Ill, 1986.

Solomon, P. "Moving from Psychoeducation to Family Education for Families of Adults with Serious Mental Illness." *Psychiatric Services,* 1996, 47, 1364–1370.

Solomon, P., Draine, J., and Delaney, M. "The Use of Restraining Orders by Families of Severely Mentally Ill Adults." *Administration and Policy in Mental Health,* 1995, 23, 157–161.

Solomon, P., Draine, J., Mannion, E., and Meisel, M. "Impact of Brief Family Psychoeducation on Self-Efficacy." *Schizophrenia Bulletin,* 1996, 22, 41–50.

Solomon, P., Draine, J., Mannion, E., and Meisel, M. "Effectiveness of Two Models of Brief Family Education: Retention of Gains by Family Members of Adults with Serious Mental Illness." *American Journal of Orthopsychiatry, 1997, 67, 177–186.*

Strachan, A. "Family Intervention for the Rehabilitation of Schizophrenia: Toward Protection and Coping." *Schizophrenia Bulletin, 1986, 12, 678–698.*

Terkelsen, K. "A Historical Perspective on Family-Provider Relationships." In H. P. Lefley and D. Johnson (eds.), *Families as Allies in Treatment of the Mentally Ill.* Washington, D.C.: American Psychiatric Press, 1990.

Vaughn, C., and Leff, J. "The Influence of Family and Social Factors on the Course of Psychiatric Illness." *British Journal of Psychiatry, 1976, 129, 125–137.*

PHYLLIS SOLOMON *is professor, University of Pennsylvania School of Social Work, and professor of social work in psychiatry, University of Pennsylvania School of Medicine.*

This chapter uses the concept of culture clash to take a fresh look at the slow progress toward family-provider collaboration. The authors discuss an intervention that targets both family culture and provider culture.

Reducing the Culture Clash in Family-Provider Relationships: A Bilateral Perspective

Edie Mannion, Marilyn Meisel

A growing core of family members, providers, and, to a lesser extent, consumers seem to agree that the ideal relationship between providers and family members in the treatment of serious mental illness is collaborative rather than hierarchical, as it has traditionally been (Bernheim, 1990; Fox, 1997; Grunebaum and Friedman, 1988; Hatfield, 1994; Intagliata, Willer, and Egri, 1986; Marsh, 1992). One rationale supporting collaboration between professional and family caregivers is that a democratic way of working facilitates better cooperation toward common goals, in contrast to the traditional, monarchical model of expecting family members to cooperate in decisions or plans that affect them, without involving them in the decision-making or planning process. Due to the consumer's right to privacy, full collaboration between families and providers requires the consumer's consent. Either the professional or a family member must proactively encourage such consent. In most cases consumers who are given an explanation of how family-provider collaboration will benefit them and their families are willing to permit at least a limited release of information to their family members. Consumer refusal to release information only partially compromises collaboration, because providers can still receive information and suggestions from family members or offer general information and support without violating confidentiality. Our combined twenty-eight years of experience in training family members and providers to work more collaboratively has convinced us that progress in family-provider relationships is occurring, but at such a slow pace that it could almost be defined as "stuck." Although the majority of both family and provider constituencies verbally support the importance of family-provider collaboration, such collaboration still seems be the exception rather than the rule. Perhaps progress can be accelerated by a new approach to this long-standing problem, a fresh paradigm for conceptualizing and improving family-provider relationships in the mental illness field. This new paradigm might come from an old concept, that of "culture clash."

Culture has been broadly defined as a shared set of values, beliefs, and behavioral norms. Culture clash results when members of one culture interact with members of a very different culture. If we assume that, despite many idiosyncratic variations among different families, the experience of loving and caring for a person who develops serious mental illness creates some common values, beliefs, and norms that reach across different cultures, socioeconomic conditions, and geographic locations, then we can loosely define families of people with mental illness as a culture. Likewise, if we also reason that choosing a career in the mental health profession, going through training, and becoming a provider of service for people with serious mental illness leads to certain common experiences that provide a core set of shared values, beliefs, and norms, then we can view providers as a culture, even though they work in different disciplines, facilities, and regions.

Support for the concept that families and providers represent two distinct cultures comes from a study of mental health professionals who have experienced mental illness in their own family, either prior to choosing a career in the mental health field or after they began their practice (Lefley, 1987). Respondents frequently commented on experiencing "cognitive dissonance because of discrepancies between etiologic concepts of family pathogenesis learned in clinical training and their observations and recollections of interactions in their own families" (p. 616). Over 90 percent of the eighty-four respondents reported that they frequently heard colleagues making negative remarks about family members, and most were not comfortable discussing the mental illness in their family with their colleagues. Their experience reflected a kind of internal conflict that is consistent with being caught in a culture clash.

Building on these assumptions, the purpose of this chapter is twofold: to compare the provider and family cultures and to endorse interventions that target both cultures in reducing culture clash and promoting collaboration. Naturally there are some overarching values shared by both groups, such as valuing the consumer's recovery and rehabilitation. One can argue that it is implausible to lump all family members together into one culture and all providers into another, due to the many variables that create subcultures within both groups. We maintain, however, that there are enough universalities in the experiences of family members and of professional care providers in our society to create a core group of values, beliefs, and norms for each group. Nevertheless, there are some subcultures within both groups whose values, beliefs, and norms vary significantly enough from one another that they warrant a distinction. Within the provider culture, for example, we have found a key distinction to be between direct service staff and administrative staff. Two primary subcultures among families of people with mental illness seem to be those who are newly exposed to the provider culture and those who have had repeated experience with it.

Understanding the Direct Service Staff Culture

First we briefly examine direct service providers' job values; attitudes and beliefs about family members; their attitudes and beliefs about their profession; and their behavioral norms in dealing with family members.

Job Values. There is wide variation in salaries among psychiatrists, psychologists, psychiatric nurses, social workers, rehabilitation counselors, case managers, and other direct service providers. If one compares the average salaries of mental health professionals to those of other professions, however, one can conclude that financial gain is not a top priority among people who choose to work in the mental health field (particularly in the public sector). What other values might drive people to choose a relatively low-paying profession? Spaniol, Jung, Zipple, and Fitzgerald (1987) have suggested that mental health professionals, like most people, value their efficacy in their jobs and believe that what they are doing is what consumers of their services want and need. Clinical training programs provide fertile soil for this professional grandiosity by emphasizing theory, interventions based on theory, and, occasionally, efficacy research, implying that consumers and families want or need the interventions taught. Functional skills assessments, needs assessments, and post-service satisfaction inventories from the client's and family's perspective are often not emphasized in training. These trends may help to explain the fact that professionals rate families as being much more satisfied with their services than do the families themselves (Hatfield, 1983; Holden and Lewine, 1982; Spaniol, Jung, Zipple, and Fitzgerald, 1987).

Although there is great variation in the goals and methods of therapeutic intervention taught in clinical training programs, both within and across disciplines, one transcending value is the importance of the therapeutic alliance between the therapist and the consumer. Many psychiatrists and therapists are trained to protect this alliance by being extremely cautious about anything that might threaten it, such as asking consumers to sign a release-of-information form that would allow some communication of information to the family. When therapists do request consent for release of information, they may ask in a way that communicates great ambivalence to the consumer and results in the withholding of consent, which then bars the therapist from disclosing information to the family. Even nonconfidential exchanges with family members can be anxiety-provoking for many professionals oriented toward treating individuals, because of their perception that such communication without the consumer's presence will jeopardize the therapeutic alliance. This perception may explain the common complaint from family members that therapists insist that the consumer be present or be told of any communication between the therapist and the family, even though this practice can lead to multiple problems for the family, the consumer, and the family-consumer relationship.

There seems to be ambivalence among professionals regarding the value of sharing power with families and consumers in making treatment decisions. Although many professionals pay lip service to the value of collaboration and empowerment inherent in the community support program philosophy, families get a different message from the behavior of many professionals. Families often report professional resistance when they request information available to the professional, question a professional's decision or judgement, assert their own values (as opposed to the professional's), or demonstrate their own knowledge or competency. Bernheim (1990) has suggested that professionals' resistance to admitting their own limitations, impotence, or ignorance, as well as their often rigid adherence to unilateral decision making, may be part of an emotional defense mechanism necessary for working within the mental illness field. The mental health care system is organized and funded in a way that requires providers to daily make numerous decisions with potentially enormous consequences, and this decision making often must occur within a context of limited time and knowledge due to inadequate funding, training, and supervision.

Attitudes and Beliefs About Family Members. The belief that poor parenting and dysfunctional families cause mental illness has been perpetuated by psychodynamic and family systems theories that lack supporting scientific evidence, and interventions based on these theories have not produced clinical improvements (Mueser and Glynn, forthcoming). Nonetheless, the former Curriculum and Training Network of the National Alliance for the Mentally Ill repeatedly found that many clinical training programs continued to teach these obsolete theories and interventions. This practice is even more harmful if students are not also exposed to critiques of these theories; to data on more effective family interventions, such as psychoeducation; or to the growing family burden literature on how mental illness adversely affects families. A subculture of providers in many facilities still holds on to the belief that families cause mental illness. Bernheim and Switalski (1988) found that up to 20 percent of the staff of a state psychiatric facility believed that mental illness is traceable to how patients are treated as children. Thirty-seven percent of the sample remained neutral, and 11 percent believed that family members of mentally ill individuals are psychologically disturbed themselves.

Provider negativity toward family members may be shifting from more obviously destructive beliefs such as family pathogenesis to more subtle forms. We have observed an increase in providers who see family members as burdened by mental illness and victimized by the mental health system. Although it is critical to acknowledge that mental illness and inadequate services have catastrophic effects on families, seeing families purely as victims is just another form of seeing them in a negative light. It can be just as difficult for professionals to form partnerships with people they perceive as victims as it is for them to work with people they perceive as villains. Providers who see families only as victims are vulnerable to difficulties in negotiating the family's responsibility in the treatment partnership and in holding families accountable when they fail to live up to responsibilities they have accepted.

Understandably, many providers have difficulty accepting the notion that they or their colleagues see families in a negative light. To break through this "not me, not us" syndrome, we start training seminars by asking providers to jot down the first thing that enters their mind when they hear the words *families of adults with mental illness*. We then show them results from past training sessions and ask them to describe those responses and compare them to their own. Over the last twelve years of doing this exercise, almost all provider responses have fallen into one of two categories: empathetic responses, such as "hopeless," "burned out," and "burdened," and more hostile responses, such as "never satisfied," "enabling," "overprotective," and even "pain in the ass." In twelve years we have seen only five responses that reflected positive attitudes toward families (for example, "caring," "coping," "strong," "love," and "support").

Beliefs About the Profession. Surveys of providers working with chronic mental illness reveal fairly high rates of burnout (Donovan, 1982; Pines and Maslach, 1978), and this may be related to providers' beliefs and attitudes about their jobs. Mirabi, Weinman, Magnetti, and Keppler (1985) found that 63 percent of public facility providers believed that the rewards of treating people with serious mental illness were unsatisfactory, and 68 percent believed that most clinicians do not receive adequate training for working with this population. Training providers to form effective working alliances with family members may partially compensate for their perceived lack of rewards and training in working with severe mental illness. However, Wright (1997) pointed out that direct service staff perceive family work as labor that is unrecognized, uncompensated, and sometimes criticized by colleagues.

Behavioral Norms in Dealing with Family Members. Involving the families of people with serious mental illness in their treatment has become a standard of good clinical practice as recognized by the Joint Commission on Accreditation of Health Care Organizations and the American Psychiatric Association. Nevertheless, family work is not routinely integrated into clinical practice (Lamb, 1990; Lehman, Thompson, Dixon, and Scott, 1995). This is the case even for family psychoeducational interventions with demonstrated clinical benefits (Dixon and Lehman, 1995). Bernheim and Switalski (1988) found that 78 percent of 350 staff members surveyed believed that families should be involved in treatment planning, but 61 percent reported spending less than one hour per week in contact with them. Less than 21 percent of 250 family members surveyed had been invited to treatment planning meetings or discharge conferences. Staff attributed this low level of family work to factors such as conflict between disciplines regarding families, time pressures, lack of experience in working with families, perceptions of confidentiality requirements, and lack of administrative support for family involvement. Wright (1997) found that staff members' attitudes toward families was not a significant factor in determining amount of family contact; rather, type of position (for example, social workers versus case managers), time of shift (day or evening), and their perception of facility efficacy had more impact.

Lefley (1988) reviewed family survey data and personal accounts (for example, Dearth, Labenski, Mott, and Pellegrini, 1986; Group for the Advancement of Psychiatry, 1986; Walsh, 1985) and concluded that the majority of providers' behavior toward families can be classified into three modes: detached, instrumental, or intrusive. In the detached mode families are avoided. The reasons for this avoidance are not explained to the families, and even when they pursue the provider, their phone calls often go unreturned. In the instrumental mode interactions are limited to those that serve the provider's needs for information, discharge planning, or financial resources to permit continuation of treatment. Discharge planning in this mode consists primarily of logistical planning rather than family preparation or education. In the intrusive mode families are invited to sessions, but the therapist's agenda takes precedence. Families' expressed needs are rarely addressed.

Understanding the Administrative Staff Culture

Valuing family involvement in treatment is not the domain of some abstract mental health "system" but the responsibility of individual program managers and administrators. Many administrators say they value family involvement; however, since financial survival is of major concern today, in the era of managed care, minimizing expensive services such as inpatient care is necessarily a top priority. Unless administrators are educated about the reductions in rehospitalization associated with certain kinds of family interventions (McFarlane and others, 1995; Solomon, Draine, Mannion, and Meisel, 1997), they may not view family inclusion in treatment as an important priority. Instead, they may continue to believe that families need only support and education that can be provided free of charge by volunteers in family support groups. Some administrators may see families as threats to consumers' confidentiality and orient their staff to carefully guard their clients' confidentiality by discouraging communication with clients' families.

Even if administrators do accept the importance of integrating family collaboration into cost-effective treatment, they may have no way to bill for the extra staff time and training required to do so. Fortunately, the mounting data on the efficacy of family interventions may soon lead managed behavioral health care organizations to reimburse providers for family work with demonstrated effectiveness. Such a shift could make family work part of the job description for certain direct service positions, rather than leaving it randomly available from providers willing to take on an "extra role."

Understanding the Culture of Families New to the Mental Health System

This section looks at families interacting with their relatives' mental health care providers for the first few times. We examine families' values regarding seeking professional help, their attitudes and beliefs about providers, their beliefs

about their relative and about themselves, and their behavioral norms in dealing with providers.

Values Regarding the Seeking of Professional Help. A family's values
concerning the seeking of professional help are largely determined by ethnic
and sociocultural variables. Serious mental illness in a loved one can be a "great
equalizer," however, and families of all cultures might eventually turn to professional providers for help for their loved ones and relief from the burdens of
caregiving. Having experienced weeks, months, or even years of coping on
their own with psychotic, regressed, suicidal, or violent behavior in their relative, most families enter the provider culture looking for a respite from their
ordeal, safety for themselves and their relative, and effective treatment that can
return their loved one to more normal functioning. Although they may value
respect, empathy, and a collaborative attitude in a provider, these values pale
in comparison with finding a provider who can offer their relative help and
hope. Families at this stage often feel intimidated and tolerate providers' negative attitudes or distressing behavior for fear that asking questions or assert-
ing themselves could have negative consequences for their ill relative.

Beliefs Regarding Providers. In this early stage families often feel overwhelmed and helpless and will initially accept a subordinate position vis-à-vis
providers they believe can help their relative. In their desperation, families may
initially believe that providers have the right to do "whatever it takes" if it will
help. Robinson and Thorn (1984) refer to this stage of professional help seeking as "naive trusting." In support of this concept, Tessler, Gamache, and Fisher
(1991) found that alienation from professionals was significantly less among
families that had only been dealing with professionals for six months.

Beliefs Regarding Their Relative and Themselves. In the early stages
of interacting with the provider culture, families may believe that their relative
has a problem, but they may not conceptualize the problem as a mental illness
(Terkelsen, 1987). They are usually not ready to believe that their relative has
a potentially serious and persistent mental illness. They may believe that someone in the family has done something to cause or worsen their relative's problem, and they may look for cues about how providers view the family's role in
the problem.

Behavioral Norms in Dealing with Providers. Understandably, families need information and emotional support when they first enter the mental
health system. The kinds of attitudes and treatment they encounter in their
early interactions with the provider culture, which often occur in emergency
rooms and inpatient settings, can be instrumental in shaping the behavioral
norms they develop in dealing with providers. Rolland (1994) calls families'
first experience with providers a "framing event" in this regard. If family members initially experience providers as empathetic, respectful, clear, and competent, the stage is set for diminished anxiety and cooperation from families.
If family members initially experience avoidant, instrumental, or intrusive
behavior from providers, they may tolerate it for a while, despite its synergis-
tic effect on their anxiety and confusion. However, continued avoidance and

exclusion from decision making, especially if there are no observable clinical improvements in their relative, gradually erode their confidence and trust in providers (Hanson, 1995; Holden and Lewine, 1982). The ending of their "naive trust" can be seen as the beginning of culture clash.

Understanding the Culture of Families Experienced with the Mental Health System

This section looks at families that have had more than a few encounters with professional providers. We examine which professional services are valued, families' attitudes and beliefs about providers, their attitudes and beliefs about themselves, and their behavioral norms in dealing with providers.

Values Concerning Professional Services. Several surveys of family self-help groups, whose members tend to have more experience with providers, indicate that their members value involvement in the treatment planning process and provision of clear information, practical advice, and emotional support from providers (Hanson, 1995; Hatfield, 1983, 1994; Holden and Lewine, 1982). Even in studies of families in which the majority did not belong to family self-help groups, information and involvement were highly valued (Bernheim and Switalski, 1988; Grella and Grusky, 1989; Spaniol, Jung, Zipple, and Fitzgerald, 1987). Mental health professionals who have experienced mental illness in their own family seem to concur with nonprofessional family members in these values (Lefley, 1987).

Attitudes and Beliefs About Providers. Family surveys have consistently shown dissatisfaction with such factors related to family-professional collaboration as provision of information and practical suggestions about mental illness, and sharing of treatment decision making (Bernheim and Switalski, 1988; Grella and Grusky, 1989; Hanson, 1995; Hatfield, 1983; Holden and Lewine, 1982; Solomon, Beck, and Gordon, 1988; Solomon and Marcenko, 1992). In our training seminars we have also tried to assess families' attitudes toward providers. We ask families, most of whom have been interacting with the mental health system for many years, to anonymously record what they first think of when they hear the term *mental health professionals*. Indications of positive associations include such responses as "working against all odds," "help," and "support." The majority of family responses have been negative, however, including remarks such as "adversarial toward family," "talk nice from two sides of their mouth," "evasive," "confusing," "lack of compassion," and "don't understand daily living with the mentally ill."

Attitudes and Beliefs About Themselves. Most studies of family experiences with mental illness indicate that families see themselves as burdened and victimized (Johnson, 1990). We have asked groups of family participants in our seminars to anonymously write down their first thoughts when they hear the phrase *families of adults with mental illness*. Responses have centered on how they have been burdened or victimized rather than how they have overcome incredible adversity. We have never received responses indicating self-perceptions of strength or resiliency. Some of the more poignant negative responses we have received include "helplessness," "desperation," "nightmare," and "end of life."

Behavioral Norms in Dealing with Providers. Families that have experienced negative attitudes or avoidant, instrumental, or intrusive behavior from providers can develop behavioral norms that are not conducive to being effective partners in treatment. These norms can include open aggression, such as making loud demands; passive aggression, such as routinely missing scheduled appointments; or sabotage of treatment, such as refusing to provide transportation, pay for further treatment, or support their relative's compliance with treatment recommendations. Conversely, it has been our experience that most families can become skilled collaborators in treatment if their relative's providers exhibit empathy and respect and provide clear information and practical suggestions regarding the illness and the mental health system.

A Bilateral Training Approach

Other authors have already suggested ways for providers to improve the quantity and quality of collaboration with family members. Hatfield (1994) has discussed ideal policies for family involvement in all types of facilities. Bernheim (1990) has presented the process used to facilitate increased family involvement in treatment teams at Buffalo Psychiatric Hospital in New York. In the area of pre-service training, members of the former Curriculum and Training Network of the National Alliance for the Mentally Ill began the process of working with directors of clinical training programs in psychiatry, psychology, psychiatric nursing, social work, and family therapy to update and improve curricula on serious mental illness and families. It is likewise important for family advocacy organizations to assume responsibility for encouraging families to develop their collaboration skills.

One promising approach with which we have been experimenting for several years is the use of collaboration seminars for family members and providers. We have been able to offer these seminars with funding from local county offices of mental health, in cooperation with local chapters of family self-help and advocacy groups or mental health associations. Leaders from all these groups can work together to plan, fund, and market such training (activities that in and of themselves promote consciousness-raising and collaboration).

Restructuring Attitudes. We have conducted these seminars with providers and family members in separate groups; with them in a single, mixed group; and with them first separated and then brought together. Written and verbal feedback from participants suggests that first training family members and providers separately and then bringing them together for a joint training experience seems to have the greatest impact on reducing their negative attitudes toward each other. Providing an opportunity for the members of each group to talk freely among themselves about their experiences with the "other culture" and then to listen to and work with members of the other group seems to strike a good balance between allowing catharsis and creating new experiences that encourage a restructuring of attitudes and beliefs. Unfortunately, logistical challenges, such as accommodating working family members who prefer evening or weekend seminars and providers who prefer weekday seminars, can make it necessary to train the two groups separately. When it is not possible to train family members and providers jointly, role-reversal exercises and personal testimonies are helpful strategies for helping these groups to empathize with each other.

Addressing Other Barriers to Collaboration. Lack of mutual empathy is just one barrier to family-provider collaboration. Bernheim (1990) and Hatfield (1994) have cited other barriers on the part of providers, such as confusion over appropriate roles for families, outdated professional ideologies, difficulty in shifting from pathology models to competency models, underdeveloped consensus-building and negotiation skills, reimbursement problems, and confidentiality issues. However, family factors, such as denial of the ill relative's chronicity or anger toward providers, also create barriers. In order to use a bilateral approach to examining barriers, we routinely ask provider and family participants in our training seminars to anonymously list their ideas about these barriers. We then collect their responses, create a master list, and hand it back to the participants on the second day of training. We keep the list of barriers identified by providers separate from the list identified by family members, so that family and provider participants can compare the two. Also, breaking down the list into domains of family variables (such as denial and poor knowledge of mental illness) and provider variables (such as lack of time, confidentiality issues, and inadequate training in working with families) helps to emphasize that both groups contribute barriers to collaboration.

The beauty of doing this exercise during joint training is that it gives everyone an opportunity to see that both groups often assign similar barriers to "the other group." For example, family members say, "Professionals lack compassion," and providers say, "Families are uncaring." Family members say, "Psychiatrists are quacks," and providers say, "Families are dysfunctional." Sometimes one group displays the very behavior they are accusing the other group of demonstrating. In one seminar the providers complained that families that do not show up for appointments do not call to cancel. We pointed out that some of their own colleagues who were registered for the training seminar never showed up or called to cancel. In many seminars family and provider participants accuse each other of avoidance, often expressing different opinions concerning whether family members or providers should initiate contact. We use these mutual accusations to demonstrate the human tendency to judge people in "other groups" for behavior one may oneself display at times. We also point out that the painful and complex human dramas brought on by mental illness may make mutual blaming a tempting coping mechanism both for families and for professional caregivers.

Opportunities for peer learning and role modeling add another ingredient to these seminars. Family members can sometimes take constructive criticism from other family members that they would not tolerate from professionals, and the same is true of providers. For example, a mother of a son with mental illness may find it easier to respect the notion that it is her responsibility to become educated about her son's illness if she hears it from another parent rather than from a professional therapist whom she perceives as having unrealistic expectations of family members. Similarly, a case manager may be less likely to insist that she does not have time to deal with her clients' families if another case manager explains the importance of making time to talk to family members.

Even when joint groups are not possible, cofacilitation of training by at least one representative of a family with a mentally ill relative, one direct service provider, and one administrator creates rich opportunities for participants to learn specific collaboration tips from others inside and outside their own culture. For example, the family member cofacilitator in one seminar commented on how much she trusts professionals who say, "I don't know" or, "I'm not sure, but I'll try to find out." The provider cofacilitator described how much it means when family members call and start the conversation with, "Is this a good time for you?" Describing, problem solving, demonstrating, and then role-playing what each individual provider and family member can do to address the barriers he or she has identified form the substance of our collaboration seminars. In one seminar a psychiatric resident described lack of knowledge about mental illness on the part of families as a major barrier. When we asked her what could be done about this barrier, she said, "Families need to be educated about mental illness." We then focused the group discussion on what she could say to a family member who lacked basic information about mental illness or where she could refer the family member for help. The group generated an excellent list of family education books and workshops as well specific suggestions about how to explain schizophrenia or mood disorders. The group also suggested that case managers receive specialized training in educating families about mental illness, since consumers and families using the public mental health system may have greater access to case managers than to office-based providers.

A common barrier to family-provider collaboration cited by providers, especially inpatient staff, is that family members are usually unavailable at the times treatment teams meet. Alternatives to having family members physically present at team meetings include options like designating one staff person as a family liaison, an approach developed by Anderson, Reiss, and Hogarty (1986). The family liaison can help ensure that the family's concerns and recommendations are heard at team meetings and that family members are kept informed about the staff's concerns and recommendations. Another alternative is telephone appointments, using conference calls and speakerphones so that more than one staff person can communicate with family members at a time.

When training family members and providers jointly, it is important to give equal time to discussion of what people in each group can do about breaking down barriers. In one joint seminar during which we were discussing time constraints, a father complained that even though his daughter signed a release-of-information form, his daughter's doctor and case manager repeatedly took many days to return his calls, allegedly due to their busy schedules. We focused the group on what he could do to overcome their time constraints. The group generated many concrete suggestions, such as making a telephone appointment at a time that would be good for the provider, preparing for the conversation by making a concise list of his questions and concerns, and disciplining himself to stick to his agenda during the conversation. We then role-played these suggestions. Brainstorming and role-playing specific suggestions replaces abstract discussions with experiential learning, which may enhance transfer of new skills to participants' own situations. Another helpful technique has been assessing people's attributions for the barriers they identify. For example, if a provider says that families' refusals to attend treatment-team meetings is a barrier, asking the provider, "Why do you think some families refuse to attend treatment-team meetings?" can help normalize behaviors that seem dysfunctional. Looking at typical family concerns, such as fear of being blamed or fear of being asked to take on more caregiving responsibility, can help providers see the adaptive features of family avoidance of treatment-team meetings. Likewise, families may be more forgiving of what they perceive as providers' shortcomings if they understand the underlying reasons for some of their practices.

Leadership. Ideally, administrators should participate in collaboration seminars, send new staff to them, and hold their staff accountable for promoting collaboration with family members. Likewise, leaders of family self-help groups should also participate in collaboration seminars, reinforce what is taught to others in their support group in such seminars, and refer new group members to collaboration training. We ask participants in our seminars to model positive attitudes and collaboration skills when they go back to their respective peer groups, either at the facilities where they work or within their families and family support groups. We propose that if every family member and provider were to take responsibility to do this, they would create a ripple effect in their respective cultures that could accelerate the breaking down of barriers to better family-provider collaboration.

Conclusion

Making family-provider collaboration a widespread practice involves large, systemwide change, but this change begins with individual attitudes. Providers, administrators, and family members must have mutual accountability for improving their attitudes about and behavior toward one another. Although many families who have had bad experiences with providers are justified in their anger, staying locked into righteous indignation about past injustice may serve to stall progress in countering stereotypes and improving providers' practices with family members. The challenge for family support and education facilitators is to help family members channel their anger and frustration into self-discipline and collaboration skills. Family members who can demonstrate to providers in a nonhostile, nonintimidating way that they have become educated (or want to become educated) about their relative's illness, want to become involved in his or her treatment, know ways of doing so without violating the confidentiality law, and can be reasonable, considerate people who make reasonable requests are taking responsibility for their role in forming collaborative relationships with providers.

On the providers' side, advocates will have to persist in challenging directors of clinical training programs to assess the values, beliefs, and norms regarding families of people with mental illness that their curricula are promoting in future providers. Administrators of provider agencies may have to take the lead in helping their staff adopt family collaboration policies and practices that conflict with their training. Administrators' biggest challenge may be overcoming staff (and, possibly, consumer) resistance to sharing decision-making power with families, especially for staff who have become comfortable with avoiding families or who see them as patients rather than partners. Overcoming staff resistance will require administrators to monitor what staff are doing to facilitate family collaboration, a task that takes a strong commitment from program managers. More studies that demonstrate the cost-effectiveness of family-provider collaboration may be the next step toward helping behavioral health care organizations make that commitment, which would then trickle down to administrators of provider agencies. In this way, managed care might offer an opportunity to overcome culture clash between families and providers.

References

Anderson, C. M., Reiss, D. J., and Hogarty, G. E. *Schizophrenia and the Family.* New York: Guilford Press, 1986.

Bernheim, K. F. "Family-Provider Relationships: Charting a New Course." In H. P. Lefley and D. L. Johnson (eds.), *Families as Allies in Treatment of the Mentally Ill.* Washington, D.C.: American Psychiatric Press, 1990.

Bernheim, K. F., and Switalski, T. "Mental Health Staff and Patients' Relatives: How They View Each Other." *Hospital and Community Psychiatry,* 1988, *39,* 63–68.

Dearth, N., Labenski, B. J., Mott, M. E., and Pellegrini, L. M. *Families Helping Families: Living with Schizophrenia.* New York: Norton, 1986.

Dixon, L., and Lehman, A. "Family Interventions for Schizophrenia." *Schizophrenia Bulletin,* 1995, *21,* 631–643.

Donovan, C. M. "Problems of Psychiatric Practice in Community Mental Health Centers." *American Journal of Psychiatry,* 1982, *139,* 456–460.

Fox, L. "A Consumer Perspective on the Family Agenda." *American Journal of Orthopsychiatry,* 1997, *67,* 249–253.

Grella, C. E., and Grusky, O. "Families of the Seriously Mentally Ill and Their Satisfaction with Services." *Hospital and Community Psychiatry,* 1989, *40,* 831–835.

Group for the Advancement of Psychiatry. *A Family Affair: Helping Families Cope with Mental Illness. A Guide for the Professions.* New York: Brunner/Mazel, 1986.

Grunebaum, H., and Friedman, H. "Building Collaborative Relationships with Families of the Mentally Ill." *Hospital and Community Psychiatry,* 1988, *39,* 1183–1187.

Hanson, J. G. "Families' Perceptions of Psychiatric Hospitalization of Relatives with a Severe Mental Illness." *Administration and Policy in Mental Health,* 1995, *22,* 531–541.

Hatfield, A. B. "What Families Want of Family Therapists." In W. McFarlane (ed.), *Family Therapy in Schizophrenia.* New York: Guilford Press, 1983.

Hatfield, A. B. "Developing Collaborative Relationships with Families." In A. B. Hatfield (ed.), *Family Interventions in Mental Illness.* New Directions for Mental Health Services, no. 62. San Francisco: Jossey-Bass, 1994.

Holden, D. F., and Lewine, R. J. "How Families Evaluate Mental Health Professionals, Resources, and Effects of Illness." *Schizophrenia Bulletin,* 1982, *8,* 626–633.

Intagliata, J., Willer, B., and Egri, G. "Role of the Family in Case Management of the Mentally Ill." *Schizophrenia Bulletin,* 1986, *12,* 699–708.

Johnson, D. L. "The Family's Experience of Living with Mental Illness." In H. P. Lefley and D. L. Johnson (eds.), *Families as Allies in Treatment of the Mentally Ill.* Washington, D.C.: American Psychiatric Press, 1990.

Lamb, H. R. "Continuing Problems Between Mental Health Professionals and Families of the Mentally Ill." In H. P. Lefley and D. L. Johnson (eds.), *Families as Allies in Treatment of the Mentally Ill.* Washington, D.C.: American Psychiatric Press, 1990.

Lefley, H. P. "Impact of Mental Illness on Families of Mental Health Professionals." *The Journal of Nervous and Mental Disease,* 1987, *175,* 613–619.

Lefley, H. P. "Training Professionals to Work with Families of Chronic Patients." *Community Mental Health Journal,* 1988, *24,* 338–357.

Lehman, A., Thompson, J., Dixon, L., and Scott, J. "Schizophrenia: Treatment Outcomes Research," *Schizophrenia Bulletin,* 1995, *21,* 561–566.

Marsh, D. *Families and Mental Illness: New Directions in Professional Practice.* New York: Praeger, 1992.

McFarlane, W. R., and others. "Psychoeducational Multiple Family Groups: Four-Year Relapse Outcome in Schizophrenia." *Family Process,* 1995, *34,* 127–144.

Mirabi, M., Weinman, M. L., Magnetti, S. M., and Keppler, K. N. "Professional Attitudes Toward the Chronic Mentally Ill." *Hospital and Community Psychiatry,* 1985, *36,* 404–405.

Mueser, K., and Glynn, S. "Family Intervention for Schizophrenia." In K. S. Dobson and K. D. Craig (eds.), *Best Practice: Developing and Promoting Empirically Validated Interventions.* Thousand Oaks, Calif.: Sage, forthcoming.

Pines, A., and Maslach, C. "Characteristics of Staff Burn-out in Mental Health Settings." *Hospital and Community Psychiatry,* 1978, *29,* 233–237.

Robinson, C. A., and Thorn, S. "Strengthening 'Family Interference.'" *Journal of Advanced Nursing,* 1984, *9,* 597–602.

Rolland, J. S. *Families, Illness, and Disability.* New York: Basic Books, 1994.

Solomon, P., Beck, S., and Gordon, B. "Family Members' Perspectives on Psychiatric Hospitalization and Discharge." *Community Mental Health Journal,* 1988, *24,* 108–117.

Solomon, P., Draine, J., Mannion, E., and Meisel, M. "Effectiveness of Two Models of Brief Family Education: Retention of Gains by Family Members of Adults with Serious Mental Illness." *American Journal of Orthopsychiatry,* 1997, *67,* 177–186.

Solomon, P., and Marcenko, M. O. "Families of Adults with Severe Mental Illness: Their Satisfaction with Inpatient and Outpatient Treatment." *Psychosocial Rehabilitation Journal,* 1992, *16,* 121–134.

Spaniol, L., Jung, H., Zipple, A. M., and Fitzgerald, S. "Families as a Resource in the Rehabilitation of the Severely Psychiatrically Disabled." In A. B. Hatfield and H. P. Lefley (eds.), *Families of the Mentally Ill: Coping and Adaptation.* New York: Guilford Press, 1987.

Terkelsen, K. G. "The Evolution of Family Responses to Mental Illness Through Time." In A. B. Hatfield and H. P. Lefley (eds.), *Families of the Mentally Ill: Coping and Adaptation.* New York: Guilford Press, 1987.

Tessler, R. C., Gamache, G. M., and Fisher, G. A. "Patterns of Contact of Patients' Families with Mental Health Professionals and Attitudes Toward Professionals." *Hospital and Community Psychiatry,* 1991, *42,* 929–934.

Walsh, M. *Schizophrenia: Straight Talk for Family and Friends.* New York: Morrow, 1985.

Wright, E. R. "The Impact of Organizational Factors on Mental Health Professionals' Involvement with Families." *Psychiatric Services,* 1997, *48,* 921–927.

EDIE MANNION is technical director of the Training and Education Center Network at the Mental Health Association of Southeastern Pennsylvania, clinical senior instructor at Allegheny University of the Health Sciences, and a therapist in private practice.

MARILYN MEISEL is executive director of the Training and Education Center Network at the Mental Health Association of Southeastern Pennsylvania and a founding member of the National Alliance for the Mentally Ill.

A peer educational program sponsored by the National Alliance for the Mentally Ill uses a unique combination of healing, consciousness-raising, and empowerment to serve long-neglected family needs.

Family-to-Family: A Trauma-and-Recovery Model of Family Education

Joyce Burland

One of the most telling indications of the failure of deinstitutionalization to improve the circumstances of individuals with serious brain disorders is the phenomenal growth of the family and consumer advocacy movement over the last twenty years. Although the early theoretical blueprints for community mental health called for alternative services designed by and for consumers and concerned family members, with both parties involved in program delivery as respected paraprofessionals, nowhere has this vision been realized in a global or systematic way. In spite of a social policy that returned seriously ill relatives to their families for care and support, traditional "blame the family" theories prevailed, and a mission to serve caring families never became an integral component of community treatment planning.

Just as nature abhors a vacuum, so do social movements abhor inertia. What the conventional wisdom of the day withholds, those whose lives and prospects hang in the balance will eventually claim. A specific case in point is family education. Over the last generation an extensive literature has developed that describes the dilemma of burden among family caregivers and suggests criteria for programs to address family needs. A number of educational curricula have been developed under the separate theoretical provinces of "psychoeducation" and "family education," and reviews of this body of work are widely available (Hatfield, 1994; Lam, 1991; Lefley, 1996; Marsh, 1992, 1994). Although appeals to provide education for families have an obvious humanitarian and practical basis, initiatives from the mental health system have been minimal to date. Outside of some university research programs and inpatient settings, along with a small number of localized programs, family education remains a scarce commodity for the thousands of caregiving families that need and deserve it.

In recent years the family caregiver movement has acted decisively to fill this void. A comprehensive family education and support program, created by combining fully developed projects of the Alliance for the Mentally Ill (AMI) of Vermont (in peer family-to-family education) and the Louisiana AMI (in peer family support group facilitation), was founded in 1992 under the Louisiana AMI trademark "Journey of Hope." In 1997 the National Alliance for the Mentally Ill (NAMI) assumed a leadership role in family education to ensure that the AMI of Vermont's family-to-family course (Burland, 1991) would continue to be offered as an integral part of NAMI's ongoing educational mission. The NAMI-sponsored family education course has been renamed "The NAMI Family-to-Family Education Program."

This chapter reports specifically on this grassroots phenomenon in family education, looking at the key features of the trauma-and-recovery approach that is the course's theoretical base. In this chapter I speak in both a personal and a collective voice to underscore the fact that although I may have shaped the family peer education program initially, it has been sustained by the many NAMI volunteers who serve as its state directors, trainers, and teachers.

Description of the Program

The NAMI Family-to-Family Education Program is a teaching model that trains family members from NAMI state affiliates to conduct a rigorous lecture and discussion course taught by co-leader pairs without professional supervision. The program was developed as an outreach service to new families in the various affiliate communities. Now going strong in many NAMI affiliates across the country, the project has grown into a full-scale national effort. At the time of this writing, hundreds of NAMI volunteers are serving as certified trained education teachers, and over twenty thousand family members have completed the full twelve weeks of classes.

The program is a self-help venture, nourished by a belief in the inherent strength of caring families and pride in the proven capabilities of NAMI family members as teachers. Here is an incredible talent pool that has been largely overlooked. In the last twenty years the family movement has matured in important ways. Largely neglected by the helping professions because of long-standing prejudice against families as the "cause" of psychiatric disorders, this group of family members of individuals with brain disorders has become one of the most advanced self-educated populations in modern medicine. This, and their lived experience at the front lines of these illnesses, qualifies them as ideal paraprofessionals in family education.

Most of the state alliances participating in the program have secured annual contracts from state departments of mental health to run it on a continuing basis. In effect they have virtually institutionalized peer family education as part of these states' community services plans. The willingness of legions of family members to serve as teachers, and their capacity to work through well-established NAMI affiliate networks across the country, mean that the family advocates' goal of universal family education may now become a reality. Here at last is the advent of a family education program that will operate in perpetuity, offered free of charge as a community service, in hundreds of towns and cities across America.

Certainly the most rewarding aspect of the family-to-family education initiative is the way families have wholeheartedly embraced it, talked about it, and referred other family members and friends to classes all over the country. In the first process evaluation of the program (Pickett, Cook, and Laris, 1997), families surveyed were overwhelmingly positive about the program. "Many respondents expressed their enthusiasm for the program with comments along the margin of their surveys, such as . . . 'this program changed my life,' . . . 'wished I had taken it years ago,' . . . 'every family should take this course!'" (pp. 27–28). Teachers report that the enthusiasm generated by the program has in many ways approached a missionary fervor in their states. It is apparent that the course has somehow sparked a response that is profoundly psychological, intensely personal, and, for many, transformative.

I wish to dwell on some of the features of the curriculum that may account for this kind of reception among families, particularly emphasizing three elements that I think are the most germane: the trauma model approach to family experience, the frank "consciousness-raising" features of the curriculum, and the forthright empowerment goals of the program. I will also note, as I go along, where this trauma-and-recovery model may differ from other models in family education.

Theoretical Basis of the Course: Secondary Intervention

The core theory behind this curriculum comes from the work of community psychiatrists Erich Lindemann (1944) and Gerald Caplan (1964). These two men, founders of the "new psychiatry" of the 1960s, declared that not everything bad that happens to people is someone's fault, that many tragic life events occur randomly and without warning, and that new models of pragmatic community treatment must assist human beings caught in the turmoil of sudden, catastrophic misfortune. Lindemann actually formulated the first secondary intervention framework for a trauma model of recovery. A review of his work finds the cornerstones of much that governs the clinical response to trauma. First, people caught in this kind of severe distress exhibit emotional reactions that are distorted but are in no way pathological; they are normative responses to frightfully abnormal circumstances. Second, people tend to adjust to such crises in normative stages; once you know what they are experiencing and what they need, you can devise anticipatory clinical interventions that will provide specific supports to help them through these stages of trauma resolution. This theoretical approach clearly honors the human capacity to surmount adversity, and its clinical genius rests on the prescription of demonstrated need as the determining factor in planning effective interventions.

Sadly, this humane clinical strategy for assisting people dealing with the capricious elements of life was rarely extended to families coping with the calamity of severe mental illness. In fact, the important theoretical distinction made by Agnes Hatfield (1994) between psychoeducation (where some putative pathology in the family must be corrected to benefit the patient) and family education (where the focus is on giving families what they need to maintain their own integrity) can be seen as a modern reflection of the dichotomy that still exists in psychiatry between primary and secondary intervention strategies for families. That is, should education be used as a tool to "treat" families as causal agents and thus prevent illness, or should education approach families in an ameliorative way to stem the cascade of secondary stressors that might further undermine their strengths as a supportive network?

The family-to-family peer program belongs securely in the second camp. It follows many of the theoretical innovations and insights provided by leading mental health professionals in NAMI who have blazed the trail to give education for the family's sake alone a respected academic base (Bernheim, 1990; Hatfield, 1990; Hatfield and Lefley, 1987; Lefley, 1996; Lefley and Johnson, 1990; Lefley and Wasow, 1994; Marsh, 1994). What this new kid on the block adds to existing theory is an avowed clinical emphasis on a trauma model of family recovery, an approach that places a high priority on family healing (as opposed to treatment), then sets this process to work—and trusts it to work—in the hands of family members themselves. Classes in the course contain all the requisite educational material covering brain disorders, and tried-and-true skill-training workshops are included as well. But the course is marked by carefully modulated exchange between educational material and the processing of the participants' traumatic feelings, and it is sustained by the high degree of sensitivity that family-member teachers bring to the realm of traumatic family experience.

Using a Trauma Model of Recovery

Combining the trauma model of recovery with family education makes enormous sense to me. Anyone who listens at length to the language of family pain will hear overtones of personal anguish as families describe their experience in the crucible of mental illness. Words like *shattering, devastating, horrendous, agony,* and *desperation* are heard repeatedly—the emotional coin of this passage. The impact of mental illness pushes family members to a level of psychic distress that goes well beyond the semantic meaning of *burden.* Families are surely loaded down with grievous and unmanageable burdens when one of their number suffers from mental illness, but they are also traumatized. By this I mean that the shock waves from this event reach to the deepest personal moorings of their lives. Trauma overwhelms people in a way that is fundamentally oppressive: it diminishes our essence while it demoralizes our spirit. To neglect this aspect of human experience in educational work with families is to miss the crucial element that, when given attention, can transform family pain into action and power.

Two contemporary psychiatrists, Judith Herman and Lenore Terr, have mapped the territory of trauma for us in ways that are exceedingly helpful. Herman (1992, p. 155) tells us that "helplessness and isolation are the core experience of trauma; empowerment and reconnection are the core experience of recovery." Psychic healing, therefore, requires three basic provisions: the establishment of safety, remembrance and mourning, and reconnection with ordinary life. To this equation Terr (1992, 1994) adds that people exposed to catastrophic life events must be led to the other side of trauma; they must be encouraged to find the meaning and significance in their suffering and helped to acknowledge the courage and sustained effort they have brought to bear in dealing with it. With this grace they can place the traumatic event into a fuller life perspective and even achieve the final psychic victory over misfortune, using the wisdom they have gained in their struggle to help others whose lives are caught in the same dire circumstances.

Teachers in the family-to-family program have come to call these emotional elements of healing "the heart of the matter," and the course is designed to provide these touchstones all along the way. Protection, privacy, and respite are paramount concerns. The program is limited to family members, with consumers attending (or teaching) only if they have a first-degree relative with a serious brain disorder. Classes are held in neutral community locations such as churches and schools rather than in mental health clinics. Basing the course on a trauma model of emotional experience means that the architecture of these classes allows family members, over the period of twelve weeks, to attain a bonding and comfort level in the group that allows them to disclose their hidden feelings of grief; break the silence they have maintained over their negative feelings of entrapment, guilt, and self-recrimination; and begin to disclose their most troubling inner thoughts.

In Class 1 the participants are immediately introduced to the stages of normative emotional reactions to trauma in a family with a mentally ill member. They are taught that their various responses to severe life dislocation are not "bad"—that each of us travels a predictable emotional path from shock and disbelief, through anger and grief, to understanding and acceptance. Finally, the course emphasizes how to place living with trauma into a life perspective that fosters self-care and self-realization.

It is absolutely certain that this focus on trauma and healing is the most appealing aspect of the course. Family members overwhelmingly endorse the emphasis on emotional self-disclosure and group affirmation of legitimate feelings, giving the highest content area score to classes focused on learning about feelings and self-care (Pickett, Cook, and Laris, 1997). Participants report that as a result of taking the course they feel more empowered, take better care of themselves, and have a happier outlook on life. They report that they feel less guilty about their relative's illness and less isolated. Many responses directly relate to the first "core experience of recovery," affirming that the course gave the participants the gift of feeling that they were not alone, that they had found a compassionate group in which to start the process of reconnection.

Using a Consciousness-Raising Technique

Let me turn to the second feature of the program that may account for families' enthusiasm for the course: its frank consciousness-raising mission. I don't
want anyone to think that we are overlooking the ill family member in this
educational venture. Reconnection between family members and their ill relative is just as crucial in a trauma model as reconnecting with others and getting on with our their lives. However, we operate from the premise that a
family's adaptation to the whole notion of mental illness begins long before
their relative becomes symptomatic. Therefore we expose families to the wide
world of stigma and discrimination to help them realize the awesome power
of negative stereotypes of mental illness and recognize how these myths can
affect the way they interpret their family member's illness and behaviors.

It is absolutely stunning to consider the avalanche of harsh messages
about mental illness that family members may have internalized. Besides the
common attributions that blame victims for bringing personal disaster upon
themselves and the hardy perennial "bad things happen to bad people," there
is the equally unforgiving code of individual responsibility; that is, if you let
yourself go, and fall apart, you deserve whatever happens to you and should
bear up without complaint. The tendency in human beings to attribute any
form of human deviance or dereliction to internal causes finds its severest
expression in attitudes toward brain disorders. Victims of these devastating illnesses are portrayed as either wanton, wicked, willful, or weak. The logical
corollary to this is family blame: anyone who raised people like this obviously
had something to do with making them turn out so badly.

Although we may advocate tirelessly to discredit these stereotypes, they
are highly intractable in the public mind, and hardly anyone remains imper-
vious to them. In the trauma model approach we take this social learning as
an unfortunate given. Families in the course refer to it as "being kept in the
dark." They are so filled with erroneous beliefs, and so much helpful information has been withheld from them because of their family association with
mental illness, that many tolerate this discrimination against them for years
without even recognizing that it exists. Whereas most family education models have the goal of correcting educational deficits in families (rather than treating their supposed character defects), we approach this matter more radically;
we call it educational *deprivation* in families due to their second-class status in
the health care system. We talk about this pointedly throughout the course to
underscore how negative stereotypes may be coloring the way families regard
their ill family member.

The most oppressive aspect of these myths is that they have persuaded
many families that mental illness is a character defect that is under their relative's control or that mental illness is incurable and so there is no hope. As a
consequence families' responses can run the gamut from inordinately high
expectations for their relatives to "snap out of it" to feelings of despair and
hopelessness because nothing can be done. Families may be most susceptible

to the myth that their ill relative can self-correct, because it implies that their loved one can be well again, fixed, with his or her potential restored, and that their agony will be over.

Therefore our primary teaching goal in this program is to liberate family members from whatever "mistaken certainties" they may have internalized about mental illness. As valid as they are for other models of family education, we don't set a priority on the learning goals of high motivation, ability to transfer learning, or long-term retention (although we do provide a handout notebook that participants build during the course and keep as a reference). We see our task as one of marshalling educational information to disconfirm and discredit every prejudice that may be preventing family members from objectifying their relative's illness and seeing it clearly as a no-fault condition. Consciousness-raising in this manner is like a teach-in: you overload the participants with information so that the accumulated weight of fact after fact will eventually break through deeply conditioned defenses. The twelve classes in the program offer a torrent of information. Teachers lecture from a uniform text that is updated annually, and over 250 pages of detailed handouts end up in participants' class notebooks.

Families actually handle this information overload very well. Many of them tell us they come to "see the light." I keep a collection of comments like these from course evaluations: "I was so pathetically in the dark about mental illness." "Why hasn't someone told me all this before?" "Without this course we would have stayed unconscious." Not only do families begin to recognize the gross misappropriation of their own lived experience, they also gain a genuine appreciation of the hardships borne by their ill relative. The shift in family members' consciousness somehow changes how they interpret behavior and allows them to empathize more fully with their relative's predicament. They write that they feel renewed in their capacity as caregivers and bolder in their dealings with the system. Families also report that "they get along better with their ill relative and have more realistic expectations about what he or she can and cannot do" and emphasize that the course is "about the process—the growth they experienced personally in understanding and coping with their loved one's mental illness" (Pickett, Cook, and Laris, 1997, p. 22).

Family Education as an Empowerment Tool

One of the themes heard repeatedly from course participants is their feelings of shock and frustration as they try to cope with deficits in the system of care for individuals with serious brain disorders. Families in need perceive very quickly that their experience would be altogether different if their stricken relative were struggling with any other legitimate illness. None could possibly imagine people with heart disease or cancer, and their families, being subjected to the systematic disregard of family caregivers that can occur when a brain disorder strikes. The privacy of the course's setting allows participants to vent these grievances fully to their peers, allowing the group to begin to identify the scope of change that will be necessary to improve the system of care. An entire class in the course is devoted to advocacy issues and advocacy training, and class participants new to NAMI are encouraged to join the local affiliate and to work with the organization to end the discrimination that so deeply affects their lives.

In this final prescription of empowerment, the three key elements of the Family-to-Family course curriculum can be seen to converge in an integrated theory of family treatment:

1. The final resolution of healing in the trauma model involves placing a catastrophic personal event into a fuller life perspective and using the experience to connect with others in a new and meaningful way.
2. Consciousness-raising liberates the mind from negative stereotypes and reveals what is manifestly unjust in the status quo.
3. The course's empowering call to action provides a significant way to express these newfound strengths in pursuit of constructive social and political change.

In a second study evaluating the course, Deal (1997) found that the most significant gains reported by class participants were on the measure of empowerment. Deal comments that from a broader, theoretical perspective, helping to empower families may be a more effective means of alleviating family burden than using traditional therapeutic interventions (p. 37). Lefley, (1992, p. 597) has made the same theoretical point, stating that "real therapy for families may well lie in their potential for mastery over the conditions that have diminished their lives." As a matter of current record, states offering the program report that over 75 percent of new family members taking the course join NAMI, and many move into leadership roles within their local and state affiliates.

In closing, let me emphasize again that this course was designed expressly for NAMI family-member teachers, and it is to their eternal credit that the program has met with such success. These volunteers have literally defined the standard for paraprofessional service in family education with their inimitable value to families as outstanding role models; their capacity to co-lead and run classes smoothly and effectively; their ability to keep a hugely detailed course on track while meeting individual class members' needs; their vast contribution of time and focused attention in conducting home visits prior to the course and in preparing for each class; their willingness to disclose the most traumatic aspects of their own experience to encourage others to "speak pain" and come through it; their humor, wisdom, and honesty; their abiding empathy for the families attending their classes; their helpfulness in connecting class participants to needed services and resources; and their kindness in serving as mentors to group members who indicate their readiness to become advocates in the family movement.

It appears that the NAMI Family-to-Family Education Program answers many family needs and offers families a dimension of healing that is long overdue. Taking families through traumatic feelings and providing them with a circle of common cause to challenge discrimination is a job that NAMI family members do with tremendous skill and dedication.

References

Bernheim, K. F. "Principles of Professional and Family Collaboration." *Hospital and Community Psychiatry,* 1990, *41,* 1353–1355.

Burland, J. C. "The AMI-Vermont Family Education Course." Brattleboro, Vt.: The Alliance for the Mentally Ill of Vermont, 1991.

Caplan, G. *Principles of Preventive Psychiatry.* New York: Basic Books, 1964.

Deal, W. P. "Evaluation of a Family Education Program for Caregivers of Individuals with Serious Mental Illness." Unpublished doctoral dissertation, Department of Psychology, University of Mississippi, 1997.

Hatfield, A. B. *Family Education in Mental Illness.* New York: Guilford Press, 1990.

Hatfield, A. B. "Family Education: Theory and Practice." In A. B. Hatfield (ed.), *Family Interventions in Mental Illness.* New Directions for Mental Health Services, no. 62. San Francisco: Jossey-Bass, 1994.

Hatfield, A. B., and Lefley, H. P. (eds.). *Families of the Mentally Ill: Coping and Adaptation.* New York: Guilford Press, 1987.

Herman, J. L. *Trauma and Recovery.* New York: Basic Books, 1992.

Lam, D. H. "Psychosocial Family Interventions in Schizophrenia: A Review of Empirical Studies." *Psychological Medicine,* 1991, *21,* 423–441.

Lefley, H. P. "Expressed Emotion: Conceptual, Clinical, and Social Policy Issues." *Hospital and Community Psychiatry,* 1992, *43,* 591–598.

Lefley, H. P. *Family Caregiving in Mental Illness.* Thousand Oaks, Calif.: Sage, 1996.

Lefley, H. P., and Johnson, D. L. (eds.), *Families as Allies in Treatment of the Mentally Ill.* Washington, D.C.: American Psychiatric Press, 1990.

Lefley, H. P., and Wasow, M. (eds.), *Helping Families Cope with Mental Illness.* Newark, N.J.: Harwood Academic, 1994.

Lindemann, E. "Symptomatology and Management of Acute Grief." *American Journal of Psychiatry,* 1944, *101,* 141–148.

Marsh, D. T. *Families and Mental Illness: New Directions in Professional Practice.* New York: Praeger, 1992.

Marsh, D. T. (ed.), *New Directions in the Psychological Treatment of Serious Mental Illness.* New York: Praeger, 1994.

Pickett, S. A., Cook, J. A., and Laris, A. *The Journey of Hope: Final Evaluation Report.* Chicago: National Research and Training Center on Psychiatric Disability, University of Illinois, 1997.

Terr, L. C. "Mini-Marathon Groups: Psychological 'First Aid' Following Disasters." *Bulletin of the Menninger Clinic,* 1992, *56* (1), 76–86.

Terr, L. C. *Unchained Memories.* New York: Basic Books, 1994.

JOYCE BURLAND is a clinical psychologist and national director of the NAMI Family-to-Family Education Program.

PART TWO

The Ethnocultural Context of the Family Experience

There is growing attention to the roles of families as caregivers of relatives with serious mental illness. This chapter examines the experiences of family caregivers in diverse cultures and discusses the implications of these experiences for the goal of supporting families in these roles.

Multicultural Experiences of Family Caregiving: A Study of African American, European American, and Hispanic American Families

Peter J. Guarnaccia

This chapter discusses findings from a study of experiences of mental illness among families from three different cultures. It describes these different cultures' experiences with U.S. mental health care resources and the unique burdens they each face in caring for an ill family member. The study was a comparative investigation of Hispanic American (primarily Puerto Rican and Cuban American), African American (including West Indian), and European American (primarily from southern and eastern Europe) families. The goal of the study was to better understand each family's perspective on caring for a seriously mentally ill family member and to learn how the family's culture influenced their recognition of symptoms, their labeling of the illness, and their responses to the family member's behavior. Through understanding these aspects of family caregiving, providers will be more able to reach out to families from a variety of cultural backgrounds and address their needs.

Researchers have only recently begun to focus on the roles minority families play in initiating and continuing treatment for the seriously mentally ill (Guarnaccia and others, 1992; Guarnaccia and Parra, 1996; Milstein, Guarnaccia, and Midlarsky, 1995; Pickett, Vraniak, Cook, and Cohler, 1993; Steuve, Vine, and Streuning, 1997). Lefley (1987a, 1990) reports that minority families view and cope with a mentally ill relative differently than European American families. Existing research indicates that pathways to treatment are affected by family members' interpretations of the patient's symptoms (Lin and Lin, 1978; Lin, Inui, Kleinman, and Womack, 1982; Rogler and Cortes, 1993).

However, few studies have explored the processes of symptom interpretation and illness definition among minority families, whose cultural construction of mental illness often deviates significantly from the cultural constructions of the majority and of professionals (Jenkins 1988, 1993; Jenkins and Karno, 1992; Guarnaccia and others, 1992).

There has been limited research in the United States on the particular burdens experienced by the families of minority patients—families whose coping capacities may be strained to the limit by scarce financial resources and fragmented community structures (Lefley 1990; Horwitz and Reinhard, 1995; Guarnaccia and Parra, 1996; Steuve, Vine, and Streuning, 1997). How such stressors affect the willingness and ability of families to provide support to patients in community treatment is a subject that has been similarly neglected. Ethnicity and social class simultaneously affect contact by both patients and families with the mental health care system, the level of family support, and the social adjustment of ill individuals in the community. The family's cultural background and social class influence how the patient, the family, and mental health professionals perceive the illness and formulate strategies for managing it (Neighbors, 1986; Boyd-Franklin and Shenouda, 1990).

Family practitioners need to understand cultural differences in the ways people conceptualize mental disorders (Edgerton and Karno, 1971; Hall and Tucker, 1985; Jenkins, 1988; Guarnaccia and others, 1992; Milstein, Guarnaccia, and Midlarsky, 1995). All families, when faced with an ill family member, try to create an understanding for themselves of what this change in their relative is and to figure out how to respond to it (Terkelsen, 1987). Cultural factors are fundamentally salient in determining how family members conceptualize their relative's abnormal behavior (Lefley, 1990; Jenkins, 1988), and the outcome of this process will be integral in the subsequent care-seeking behavior of family members. For practitioners to communicate effectively with families they must fully understand the cultural assumptions of the persons to whom they are speaking.

How families seek mental health services for their family members and the pathways they follow into treatment are subjects that have received renewed attention. Pathways into mental health treatment are defined as the sequence of contacts with individuals and agencies that are prompted by a distressed person's efforts, and those of their relatives or significant others, to seek help, as well as the help that is supplied in response to such efforts (Lin and Lin, 1978; Lin, Inui, Kleinman, and Womack, 1982; Rogler and Cortes, 1993). The importance of understanding the pathways to treatment that individuals in a given family follow is that doing so can uncover the critical link between the onset of psychiatric difficulties and the unique, socioculturally driven way in which families utilize the mental health care system. In the literature regarding help seeking, the culturally distinct features of African American and Latino families, compared to their European American counterparts, include denser support networks and exposure to more informal helping agents; diverse and varying conceptions of mental illness, which influence these families' sensitivity to stigmatization; and differing degrees of family burden. These differences among families of different cultures are prominent in certain patterns of help seeking.

Profile of the Families

The observations discussed in this chapter are from interviews with the main caregiving family member of persons with serious mental illness. The families were identified through family groups and client populations of public community mental health centers and state psychiatric hospitals in the state of New Jersey. The sample consisted of individuals with family members whose course of mental illness was prolonged and who required significant functional and emotional support from their families over an extended period. The relationship of the people interviewed to the mentally ill individual included parent, spouse, adult sibling, and adult child. For the most part the psychiatric diagnoses of the ill individuals, as reported by the families and the clinical staff, were schizophrenia, bipolar disorder, or major depression.

The study consisted of in-depth interviews with the family member who identified herself or himself as being most involved in caring for the ill individual. The objective of these interviews was to determine how the family members responded to and coped with the patients' illness. The interviews lasted approximately one and a half hours and covered the family's overall experience with the mental health care system, their conception of the problem, their social support systems, and the problems they experienced as a result of having a relative with mental illness.

It is important to emphasize that this was an exploratory study and that the sample was an opportunistic one. Caution needs to be taken in generalizing from this sample to the larger groups reflected by it. In this chapter I highlight areas of commonality and large differences between the ethnic groups involved.

Social Characteristics of the Families. Half of the ninety families interviewed were Hispanic American: thirty of these were Puerto Rican, six were Cuban American, and nine were families from Central or South America. One-third of the families were African American, and 18 percent were European American.

Many of the primary caregivers were parents, and their main concern was what would happen to their adult child when they were no longer able to take care of him or her. The issue of aging caregivers has become a national concern among advocates for families of the mentally ill (Lefley, 1987b). The average age of the caregivers, by ethnic group, was forty-eight for the Hispanic Americans, fifty-four for the African Americans, and fifty-five for the European Americans. The average age of the ill family member, again by ethnic group, was forty, thirty-four, and thirty-five, respectively. The younger age of the Hispanic caregivers and the older age of their ill family members is largely due to the unique presence of married couples among the Hispanics, where one spouse was the caregiver and the other the ill family member (see Table 4.1).

Table 4.1. Social Characteristics of Main Caregivers

Social Characteristics	Hispanic (percent)	African American (percent)	European American (percent)
Age (mean)	48	54	55
Gender			
Female	80%	90%	87%
Male	20	10	13
Relationship to ill relative			
Parent	42	76	75***
Daughter/son	20	3	0
Spouse	22	0	6
Sibling	13	21	19
Education			
Elementary or less	46	7	6***
Some high school	27	14	0
High school diploma or higher	27	79	94
Family income			
$9,999 or less	41	18	7
$10,000–$19,999	37	18	13
$20,000–$29,999	18	14	27
$30,000–$39,999	2	18	13
$40,000+	2	32	40
Household composition			
Dual parent/extended family	67	38	69**
Female head	33	62	31
N = 90	n = 45	n = 29	n = 16

Chi-square **$p < .01$, ***$p < .001$.

Mothers were the most frequent caregivers. Forty-eight percent were mothers, and another 30 percent were sisters, daughters, wives, or other female relatives. In 80 percent of the cases the everyday care of the mentally ill family member was in the hands of a woman relative. The feminization of the care of individuals with mental illness is another key issue in working with families (Cook, 1988). When the woman is herself working and caring for other family members, she experiences multiple burdens related to caring for an ill relative. These problems are made more severe when the woman caregiver is a single head of household. Further complications occur for female caregivers when the ill relative is a son or brother who becomes aggressive or violent during periods of worsening symptoms. These problems call for special support systems for these families.

The African American households were less likely than the Hispanic American or the European American households to contain both parents. Two-thirds of the African American households were headed by women, compared to one-third of the Hispanic American households and one-quarter of the European American households. European American caregivers, often siblings of the ill family member, were the only caregivers to report that they lived alone. These findings indicate the need for additional adult support people, either other family or friends, to assist these primary caregivers of mentally ill family members. Although European Americans have found these supports, to some extent, through family groups such as the Alliances for the Mentally Ill, minority families rely on informal networks of kin and friends and use formal support groups less often. New models for building supports for minority caregivers are needed.

Household income was calculated by aggregating all sources of income, including social security income and welfare benefits. Of the three groups, the Hispanic Americans were the poorest. Seventy-eight percent of the Hispanic families reported a total annual income of less than $20,000, and of these 41 percent reported less than $10,000. This finding is particularly striking since the majority of Hispanic households had at least one employed member. In our sample, almost 65 percent of the African American families and 90 percent of the European American families reported incomes of more than $20,000. Forty percent of the European American families had annual incomes of $40,000 or more. In spite of the range of incomes of the families in our study, most of the families were dependent on public mental health services and reported that limited incomes led to fewer choices in mental health services.

Social Characteristics of the Relatives with Mental Illness. The majority of the family members with mental illness were between fifteen and forty-five years old (see Table 4.2). Three-quarters of the Hispanic American and almost 60 percent of the African American ill family members lived with the primary caregiver's family; this was true for about one-third of the European American subjects. Ill individuals from European American families either lived in residential programs or lived on their own in the community. These differences reflect both the different families' preferences for where their ill family member lived and the availability of residential programs to minority families.

The families reported giving a range of help to their ill family member. They most frequently provided social and emotional support, such as being there to talk to and inviting their family member to social activities. Families also helped with meal preparation and shopping for food, taking medications and keeping clinic appointments, managing money, and doing personal chores such as laundry and self-care. Minority families tended to provide more instrumental help because their ill family members were more likely to live with them. Often families underestimated the number of things they did to help their ill family member, as they saw some of the help they provided simply as things that family members do for members still living in the household. Because the majority of the caregivers were women, many of the everyday tasks that were done for the ill family member were not seen as "work" but as part of the "normal woman's role" in the family.

Table 4.2. Social Characteristics of the Relatives with Mental Illness

Social Characteristics	Hispanic (percent)	African American (percent)	European American (percent)
Age			
29 or younger	22%	31%	38%
30–44	45	48	44
45 or older	33	21	19
Gender			
Female	51	28	25**
Male	49	72	75
Education			
Elementary or less	36	5	0***
Some high school	17	33	8
High school diploma or higher	47	62	92
Living arrangement			
Living with caregiver	78	59	31**
Living with own family	6	0	13
Living alone or in a residential program	16	41	56
Help received			
Personal grooming	43	44	27
Meal preparation and grocery shopping	66	46	40
Medical care, taking medication, keeping appointments	64	36	8***
Money management	47	54	33
Social and emotional support	98	85	80*
N = 90	n = 45	n = 29	n = 16

Chi-square *p < .05, **p < .01, ***p < .001.

Family Burden and Sources of Support for Caregivers

The minority families tended to have larger social support networks than the European American families, and these networks included more kin (see Table 4.3). The African Americans and Hispanic Americans sought out other family members for advice far more than the European Americans. The European American families turned to mental health professionals for advice more often than the minority families. This seems to be related to the differences in their respective conceptions of their family member's illness. The European Americans saw the illness more as a medical problem, whereas the minority families attributed the problem to a wider range of causes and consequently sought advice from other areas. Two of the most striking findings were that none of the European American families sought out religious advisers and that the Hispanic Americans most frequently had no one to turn to for advice (perhaps due to family isolation resulting from migration processes and to the lack of bilingual mental health professionals).

Table 4.3. Caregivers' Social Support and Areas of Problems

Supports and Problems	Hispanic (percent)	African American (percent)	European American (percent)
Size of network			
1–2	21%	35%	36%
3 or more	79	65	64
Sources of support for advice (percent yes)			
Family	38	45	27
Medical	27	17	33
Religious	2	7	0
Nobody	22	10	13
Other	11	21	27
Sources of support for concerns (percent yes)			
Family	57	59	40
Medical	2	3	0
Religious	9	3	0
Nobody	16	3	20
Other	16	31	40
Major areas of problems			
Financial burden	52	62	64
Effect on physical or mental health	52	52	93*
Disruption of family routine	74	59	87
Disruption of social life	41	18	50
N = 90	n = 45	n = 29	n = 16

Chi-square *$p < .05$.

Members of all of the families turned to other family members when they needed to talk about general concerns or to ventilate their feelings and frustrations with the burdens of caregiving. Few families turned to mental health professionals other than to talk about treatment advice. The European Americans and the Hispanic Americans were more likely than the African Americans to have no one to talk to when they needed to share their concerns about their ill family member.

All of the families saw disruption of family routine due to the inconsistent behavior of their family member as a problem. The European American families reported the greatest effects on their physical and mental health as a result of caregiving, even though the minority families were more likely to have more direct contact with their ill family member. This may be due in part to the greater limitations of the European Americans' social support networks. The European American families had smaller networks and fewer kinds of people to talk with, both for advice and for sharing concerns—resources that could enable them to vent and reduce stress as well as to receive needed help at more stressful times (Horwitz and Reinhard, 1995).

The families did not report financial burden as a primary problem connected to their caregiving. Most of the ill family members' care was paid for by public funds. In addition, most of the ill family members received some form of income support. The income support was often crucial in allowing families to continue to care for their ill family member at home. These social security programs, including medical insurance and income support, are especially vital to maintaining minority and low-income individuals in care and in the community. The financial burdens reported in Table 4.3 seem to reflect limitations on working outside the home due to the time constraints of taking care of an ill family member rather than direct financial problems caused by paying for the family member's care. Many families did express frustration that their choice of services and treatment options was limited by their lack of financial resources, however.

Many families did not see caring for their family member only as a burden; many viewed caregiving as both rewarding and stressful (Greenberg, Greenley, and Benedict, 1994). For most of the family caregivers, tasks such as cooking, doing laundry, and managing money were seen as just part of what you do for family. This was particularly true for the African American and Hispanic American families. The families did report the need for respite care to help them when they felt overwhelmed or wanted to get away for a few hours or days.

The Families' Conceptions of the Illness

The families were asked to describe the kind of problem they thought their family member had (see Table 4.4). The responses to this question were recoded into four categories. "Medical" responses included descriptions of the problem as a chemical imbalance or other type of brain problem. "Emotional" responses focused on problems of nervousness; among the Hispanic families this was summarized in the cultural concept of *nervios* (Guarnaccia and Farias, 1988; Jenkins, 1988). Families who described their ill member's problem using personality descriptors like "selfish" or "aggressive" were placed in the "Personality" category. The final category was "Social," which included those who discussed the problem in terms of interacting with others or problems in relationships. The Hispanic families tended to feel strongly that their relative was suffering from a problem that was more emotional than medical. The European Americans and the African Americans reported in equal numbers that they felt their relative was suffering from a problem that was medical in nature; in both of these groups this was the most frequent response. The African American and European American families were also more likely to perceive their family member's problem as stemming from negative personality traits than were the Hispanic families. The African American families were most likely of the three groups to perceive their family member's problem as one related to social interaction.

Families were also asked what professionals called their relative's problem. Schizophrenia was the most common response for all the families, particularly so for the European American families. Over one-third of the

Table 4.4. Conception and Labeling of the Illness by the Caregiver and Health Professionals

Conception of Illness	Hispanic (percent)	African American (percent)	European American (percent)
Caregiver's conception of the illness			
Medical: mental failure, chemical imbalance	20%	31%	31%*
Emotional: nervousness, anxiety	40	28	31
Personality: selfishness, aggression	4	21	19
Social: interaction with others	9	17	6
Other, don't know	27	3	13
Professional's label for illness			
Specific psychiatric label	44	64	81
General emotional or medical	20	16	6
Don't know	36	20	13
Agreement with professional's label			
Agree	39	44	77*
Expectation of Cure			
Yes	67	60	19**
N = 90	n = 45	n = 29	n = 16

Chi-square *$p < .05$, **$p < .01$.

Hispanics and one-fifth of the African American respondents did not know the diagnosis of their ill family member. This may well be an indication of differential education of families about mental illness. There are several possible explanations for these differences. For Hispanics, language barriers to obtaining information are significant, although many of the Hispanic families were recruited through agencies with Spanish-speaking staff. Some minority families may not have been told the diagnosis at all; others may have been informed about the illness in such a way that they did not retain the information. Another explanation could be that the professionals' label did not match their own view of the illness, and saying "don't know" was a polite way of rejecting the professional model.

Clear differences did emerge among the ethnic groups in the extent to which the families agreed with what the professionals indicated was the problem, with minorities disagreeing with professional assessments much more than European Americans. This lends further support to the hypothesis that some minority families actively reject professional models of mental illness. Three-quarters of the European American families agreed with the professionals' label of the illness; more strikingly, none reported that they disagreed with the diagnosis. African Americans reported more disagreement than Hispanics, whereas Hispanics more often responded that they did not know the diagnosis. This result may reflect greater distrust of professionals by African Americans and a greater deference to authority by Hispanics (Boyd-Franklin and Shenouda, 1990; Garcia-Preto, 1982; Jones and Gray, 1986).

One of the most striking interethnic differences was in the area of expectation of a cure. The Hispanics and African Americans expressed much stronger expectations that their family member's illness would be cured than did the European Americans. This difference may result, in part, from the greater involvement with and effectiveness of psychoeducation approaches with European American families (McFarlane, 1983; Falloon, Boyd, and McGill, 1984). Strong religious beliefs in the healing power of God are another factor affecting these different perceptions; these beliefs were more strongly expressed by minority families. A need for further understanding of the different meanings of *cure* across groups and the role of optimism in caregiving is suggested by these results (Milstein, Guarnaccia, and Midlarsky, 1995).

Pathways to Care

There were significant differences in the pathways to care taken by the African American and the European American families. Employing models developed by Lin and others (Lin and Lin 1978; Lin, Inui, Kleinman, and Womack, 1982), we observed the following patterns of help seeking (see Table 4.5). In the first hospitalization (Pathway 1), African Americans demonstrated much more family involvement, culturally based resource use, community leader consultation, and reluctance in accepting psychiatric referral (Pathway Type A) in their response to their family member's mental illness. During their first hospitalization, African Americans followed Pathway Type A 47 percent of the time, whereas European Americans followed this pathway only 13 percent of the time. In contrast, European Americans were much more likely to seek help from a mental health professional early on and demonstrated multiple contacts with and frequent utilization of formal agencies (Pathway Type B). The predominant pathway to the first hospitalization for European Americans was Type B (73 percent), whereas African Americans followed this pathway much less frequently (30 percent). Additionally, in Pathway 1 there was a greater amount of legal and social agency involvement (Pathway Type C) in the African Americans' help-seeking experience (23 percent) than was seen in the European Americans' overall utilization pattern (13 percent), although this was not the predominant pathway type for either group.

The patterns of utilization continued to be significantly different in the most recent hospitalization discussed in the interview (Pathway 2). In Pathway 2, Pathway Type A was experienced 56 percent of the time by the African American families, compared to only 8 percent for the European Americans. Pathway Type B was followed 61 percent of the time by the European American families, in contrast to 22 percent for the African Americans. There was a shift in Pathway Type C utilization for this hospitalization period, with the European Americans showing an increase in this pathway type (31 percent) and the African Americans continuing to follow Pathway Type C at rates similar to the first hospitalization (22 percent). With the exception of one African

Table 4.5. Ethnicity and Pathways to Care

Pathway Type	African American	European American
1. First Hospitalization		
Type A	14 (47%)	2 (13%)
Type B	9 (30%)	11 (73%)
Type C	7 (23%)	2 (13%)**
N = 45	n = 30	n = 15
2. Most Recent Hospitalization		
Type A	13 (56%)	1 (8%)
Type B	5 (22%)	8 (61%)
Type C	5 (22%)	2 (31%)**
N = 34	n = 23	n = 11

Chi-square **$p < .01$.

American family for which the school intervened in seeking treatment, all of the families who utilized Type C pathways involved police interventions.

Implications for Working with Families

This study was designed to provide a profile of the experiences of caregiver families from different ethnic groups. What clearly emerges from the study are the central roles of culture, ethnicity, and social status in shaping families' experiences of caregiving. With the continuing trend of downsizing and closing state psychiatric hospitals, families will increasingly play a major role in the care of the seriously mentally ill. Given the overrepresentation of minorities in the public mental health system, a fuller understanding of minority families' experiences, both with their ill family member and with the mental health system, is needed. Several issues for practitioners working with families of various cultures are raised by this chapter.

A central issue is differences both between and within ethnic groups in definition of the family, its perceived role in caregiving, and normative patterns of family growth and development. Our study suggests that Hispanics and African Americans maintain closer family ties both with adult children and with other relatives. This is by no means a new finding, but its implications for family caregiving for the seriously mentally ill are only beginning to be explored. Also, minority families are much more likely to expect unmarried family members to remain at home, regardless of their health, and are more likely to feel a strong obligation and preference for caring for seriously ill family members at home.

Differing definitions of and values placed on autonomy and independence by different ethnic groups play a key role in family responses to a mentally ill family member. The general approach of mental health professionals is to see client independence and autonomy as the ultimate goal. Much of the literature on family emotional environments focuses on the negative impacts of overinvolvement (Jenkins, 1993). Across cultures, families differ markedly in their values concerning family interconnectedness and involvement. Particularly in the case of serious mental illness, families from many cultural groups see it as the responsibility of the family to care for the individual, and suggestions that the family should become less involved or that the ill individual should live outside the family home are viewed as challenges to the integrity of the family.

An important issue related to definitions of the family is the assessment of family burden. Much of the focus of recent research on families of the mentally ill has been on burden, and this has been an appropriate corrective to earlier views that blamed families for the mental illness of their family member. However, less attention has been paid to balancing research on burdens with examination of the rewards of caregiving and reciprocal aid between mentally ill individuals and their caregivers, who are often elderly adults (Greenberg, Greenley, and Benedict, 1994). In understanding what leads caregivers to remain involved with their ill family member or to disconnect from him or her, this more balanced view may provide additional insights. Also, the more family members see caregiving as part of what you do for family, the less likely they are to accurately provide information on their caregiving tasks and burdens. We found that we needed to be fairly detailed in asking about the range of help the families provided, because they saw many of these supports as a normal part of what they do for family and did not have in mind some economic calculus. They did not think about the fact that if they did not provide these services, some social agency would have to do it.

Also related to these issues are needs for better methods of assessing the social supports available to seriously mentally ill individuals and their families and for more innovative ways to provide supports to families of various different cultures. There is a need for additional family support models to complement the very effective approach the National Alliance for the Mentally Ill (NAMI) has developed among European American families. Given the expressed need by families in our study for groups that provide information and support yet the very low involvement of minority families in NAMI groups and in various formal psychoeducational programs, an important research agenda is identifying and assessing alternative models. Although cross-cultural researchers have examined the role of social networks based on churches and other community supports, findings from these studies have become central neither to mental health services research nor to family program development.

Two of the most frequently discussed concerns and points of dissatisfaction among the families was their need for more information about their family member's illness and their need to know where to go for help. This "need to know" for families with a mentally ill family member has been elucidated by Hatfield (1987). She points out that families need clear, nontechnical explanations about their family member's illness. In addition, they need advice concerning appropriate expectations, specific techniques for managing difficult behavior, and the availability of community resources. Although NAMI has been very effective in advocating for and developing such programs for European American families, these kinds of programs are still not widely accessible to African American and Hispanic families. The caregiver's conception of the illness can play a critical role in the interaction between family members and professionals. If, for example, caregivers have a divergent conceptualization of their family member's illness from that of the professional, a schism can occur, creating strained or even absent communication between caregiver and professional. This communication is necessary, however, so that the caregiver will have knowledge about ongoing treatment, the course and severity of the illness, what to do, and what to expect (Terkelsen, 1987). Consequently, differences in illness conception, as well as many other negative experiences that shape caregivers' level of service satisfaction, can lead to further estrangement from mental health professionals. This lack of communication can result in further limiting of caregivers' access to vital information concerning the care of their ill family member.

In terms of access to services, several additional issues emerge when minority families are included in studies. The issue of language barriers for Hispanic and other non-English-speaking families looms large. Language barriers affect access to information about mental illness and services to treat it, determine how effectively crises are reported and managed, structure the range of services available to clients and families, shape the diagnostic and therapeutic processes, and determine the availability and suitability of posthospitalization resources. Discrimination and racism on the part of the system and individual providers also shape the clinical process—in our study this problem was strongly suggested by the lower involvement of African American individuals in therapeutic interventions. Another area where these issues emerge is in assessing the appropriateness of police intervention. Although the ill person's behavior is certainly a major determinant in this area, more research is needed to establish that the greater involvement of police in the hospitalizations of African Americans is not based on discriminatory judgments of the threat posed by individuals from different ethnic groups.

Cultural issues also appear to affect the accessibility and acceptability of a variety of supportive services for the mentally ill. There is continuing controversy about whether minority clients in the mental health system should be served using different models of care or whether current models need to better accommodate minority individuals (Rodriguez, Lessinger, and Guarnaccia, 1992). One issue is the lack of developed models of culturally competent day treatment programs, vocational rehabilitation programs, and family psychoeducation programs to compare to more standard programs (Rivera, 1988). This is clearly a precursor to needed research on the relative effectiveness of ethnic-group-accommodated versus ethnic-group-specific services for the seriously mentally ill.

An overwhelming majority of the families we interviewed identified the following as major areas of need. Vocational rehabilitation and training programs were a high priority for the majority of the families, for at least two reasons: they provide structured activity, which increases self-esteem, and they address some of the families' concerns about the future of the ill family member. Family members expressed a need for more social contacts and activities (especially on weekends) for their ill relatives in which they could interact with peers who share similar problems. Several families also suggested some kind of companion program for their ill family member. The families were concerned about the availability and quality of residential options for their family members. Although there were marked differences between families of different cultural and social class backgrounds concerning where they felt their ill family member should live at present, all the families were concerned about housing options for the future. Family members wanted assistance with future planning, especially in terms of planning for who will care for the ill family member when the current caregiver is no longer able to provide support and where the ill family member will live.

Several respondents' conceptions of their family member's problem were not shaped by the medical model of schizophrenia (the most common diagnosis). The extent of this divergence appeared especially prominent among minority families. Religious belief and social class also played important roles in shaping the families' conceptions of mental illness. This is an important area for more education. It is important to explore families' ideas about mental illness and to take their conceptions into consideration before explaining schizophrenia or other forms of psychiatric disorder. The need for multiple models of family psychoeducation that are sensitive to social and cultural differences is critical.

A major form of help for families of the mentally ill has been the development of psychoeducation programs that focus on educating families about serious mental illness and its treatment, helping families develop methods for coping with problematic behaviors, and building support networks among families with a mentally ill family member (Falloon, Boyd, and McGill, 1984; McFarlane, 1983; Rivera, 1988). Rivera (1988) presented an assessment of the applicability of the psychoeducation model to Hispanic families, using her experience with a family support group in the Bronx. Rivera argued that the inclusion of families in treatment, the focus on providing concrete information about mental illness, the use of concrete treatments such as medications and explicit behavioral instructions, and the effort to alleviate families' sense of shame over the illness were all compatible with Hispanic culture and fit with the needs identified by Hispanic families in the Bronx. At the same time, she argued that the use of an egalitarian problem-solving paradigm within psychoeducation, the lack of attention to spiritual factors in illness, the misinterpretation of some spiritual beliefs as signs of psychosis, and the problematic assessment of what constitutes overinvolvement with an ill family member all suggest the need to modify the psychoeducational approach in using it with Hispanic families.

This chapter has provided further insights into the ways family educational programs need to be modified for families from different cultures. Many families' conceptions of mental illness are rooted in cultural models that see mental illness as a continuum. These ideas about illness allow families both to be accepting of their family member and to maintain some hope for the future. Introducing information to families about the medical model of schizophrenia and other serious mental illness needs to be done in a way that acknowledges and builds on their conceptions. At a minimum, educational programs need to start by assessing families' understandings of mental illness and working from those ideas. A more difficult task will be to come to terms with the implications of the medical model for different families' acceptance of and hope for their ill family member. I am not advocating that families not be provided the most current medical information on their family member's disorders; rather, I am arguing that any model of illness carries with it value judgements about the person and expectations for his or her future. These issues need to be discussed openly with providers and among families. In order to achieve this goal, providers need to develop a deeper understanding of culturally diverse families' perspectives on mental illness and the implications of these perspectives for their role as caretakers.

A second assumption of family education models is that families are isolated from their natural support networks by mental illness, so a new network—of families with mentally ill members—needs to be created. This model has, in fact, worked quite well with European American families. Many of the African American and Hispanic families in our study had much broader social networks and did not experience the ruptures with relatives and friends that the European American families experienced. Many of the minority families' social networks provided significant support. This suggests that family models can and need to build on the strengths of this social and cultural matrix within minority communities in designing family intervention models. Psychoeducation groups for these communities, rather than being built on groups of unrelated individuals or couples who share a similar problem, might be built on larger family networks that share ties of kinship or membership in key community institutions such as churches. Mental health professionals need to develop a culturally integrative approach to working with families that respects their salient cultural conceptions of mental illness at the same time that it provides additional treatment information.

References

Boyd-Franklin, N., and Shenouda, N. T. "A Multisystems Approach to the Treatment of a Black, Inner-City Family with a Schizophrenic Mother." *American Journal of Orthopsychiatry,* 1990, *60,* 186–195.

Cook, J. A. "Who 'Mothers' the Chronically Mentally Ill?" *Family Relations,* 1988, *37,* 42–49.

Edgerton, R., and Karno, M. "Mexican-American Bilingualism and the Perception of Mental Illness." *Archives of General Psychiatry,* 1971, *224,* 286–290.

Falloon, I.R.H., Boyd, J., and McGill, C. *Family Care of Schizophrenia.* New York: Guilford Press, 1984.

Garcia-Preto, N. "Puerto Rican Families." In M. McGoldrick, J. Pearce, and J. Giordano (eds.), *Ethnicity and Family Therapy.* New York: Guilford Press, 1982.

Greenberg, J. S., Greenley, J. R., and Benedict, P. "Contributions of Persons with Serious Mental Illness to Their Families." *Hospital and Community Psychiatry*, 1994, *45*, 475–480.

Guarnaccia, P. J., and Farias, P. "The Social Meanings of *Nervios*: A Case Study of a Central American Woman." *Social Science and Medicine*, 1988, *26*, 1223–1231.

Guarnaccia, P. J., and Parra, P. "Ethnicity, Social Status and Families' Experiences of Caring for a Mentally Ill Family Member." *Community Mental Health Journal*, 1996, *32*, 243–260.

Guarnaccia, P. J., and others. "*Si Dios Quiere*: Hispanic Families' Experiences of Caring for a Seriously Mentally Ill Family Member." *Culture, Medicine and Psychiatry*, 1992, *16*, 187–215.

Hall, L., and Tucker, C. "Relationships Between Ethnicity, Conceptions of Mental Illness, and Attitudes Associated with Seeking Psychological Help." *Psychological Reports*, 1985, *57*, 907–916.

Hatfield, A. B. "Families as Caregivers: A Historical Perspective." In A. B. Hatfield and H. P. Lefley (eds.), *Families of the Mentally Ill: Coping and Adaptation*. New York: Guilford Press, 1987.

Horwitz, A., and Reinhard, S. "Ethnic Differences in Caregiving Duties and Burdens Among Parents and Siblings of Persons with Severe Mental Illness." *Journal of Health and Social Behavior*, 1995, *36*, 138–150.

Jenkins, J. "Conceptions of Schizophrenia as a Problem of Nerves: A Cross-Cultural Comparison of Mexican-Americans and Anglo-Americans." *Social Science and Medicine*, 1988, *26*, 1233–1243.

Jenkins, J. "Too Close for Comfort: Schizophrenia and Emotional Overinvolvement Among Mexicano Families." In A. D. Gaines (ed.), *Ethnopsychiatry*. Albany: State University of New York Press, 1993.

Jenkins, J., and Karno, M. "The Meaning of Expressed Emotion: Theoretical Issues Raised by Cross-Cultural Research." *American Journal of Psychiatry*, 1992, *149*, 9–21.

Jones, B. E., and Gray, B. A. "Problems in Diagnosing Schizophrenia and Affective Disorders Among Blacks." *Hospital and Community Psychiatry*, 1986, *37*, 61–65.

Lefley, H. P. "Culture and Mental Illness: The Family Role." In A. B. Hatfield and H. P. Lefley (eds.), *Families of the Mentally Ill*. New York: Guilford Press, 1987a.

Lefley, H. P. "Aging Parents as Caregivers of Mentally Ill Adult Children." *Hospital and Community Psychiatry*, 1987b, *38*, 1063–1070.

Lefley, H. P. "Culture and Chronic Mental Illness." *Hospital and Community Psychiatry*, 1990, *41*, 277–286.

Lin, K-M., Inui, T. S., Kleinman, A. M., and Womack, W. M. "Socio-cultural Determinants of the Help-Seeking Behavior of Patients with Mental Illness." *The Journal of Nervous and Mental Disease*, 1982, *170*, 78–85.

Lin, T-Y., and Lin, M-C. "Service Delivery Issues in Asian-North American Communities." *American Journal of Psychiatry*, 1978, *135*, 454–457.

McFarlane, W. (ed.), *Family Therapy in Schizophrenia*. New York: Guilford Press, 1983.

Milstein, G., Guarnaccia, P., and Midlarsky, E. "Ethnic Differences in the Interpretation of Mental Illness: Perspectives of Caregivers." In J. R. Greenley (ed.), *The Family and Mental Illness*. Research in Community and Mental Health, no. 8. Greenwich, Conn.: JAI Press, 1995.

Neighbors, H. W. "Socioeconomic Status and Psychological Distress in Adult Blacks." *American Journal of Epidemiology*, 1986, *124*, 779–793.

Pickett, S. A., Vraniak, D. A., Cook, J. A., and Cohler, B. A. "Strength in Adversity: Blacks Bear Burden Better Than Whites." *Professional Psychology: Research and Practice*, 1993, *24*, 460–467.

Rivera, C. R. "Culturally Sensitive Aftercare Services for Chronically Mentally Ill Hispanics: The Case of the Psychoeducation Treatment Model." *Hispanic Research Center Research Bulletin*, 1988, *11* (1), 1–9.

Rodriguez, O., Lessinger, H., and Guarnaccia, P. "The Societal and Organization Contexts of Culturally Sensitive Services." *Journal of Mental Health Administration*, 1992, *19*, 213–223.

Rogler, L. H., and Cortes, D. E. "Help-Seeking Pathways: A Unifying Concept in Mental Health Care." *American Journal of Psychiatry,* 1993, *150,* 554–561.

Steuve, A., Vine, P., and Streuning, E. "Perceived Burden Among Caregivers of Adults with Serious Mental Illness: Comparison of Black, Hispanic and White Families." *American Journal of Orthopsychiatry,* 1997, *67,* 199–209.

Terkelsen, K. "The Meaning of Mental Illness in the Family." In A. B. Hatfield and H. P. Lefley (eds.), *Families of the Mentally Ill.* New York: Guilford Press, 1987.

PETER J. GUARNACCIA *is associate professor of human ecology and investigator at the Institute for Health, Health Care Policy and Aging Research at Rutgers, the State University of New Jersey.*

This chapter examines the support group experiences of minority families of persons with mental illness.

Support Group Satisfaction: A Comparison of Minority and White Families

Susan A. Pickett, Judith A. Cook, Tamar Heller

Support groups have become an increasingly important resource for families of persons with mental illness. These groups, which may be led by other family members through organizations such as the National Alliance for the Mentally Ill (NAMI) and the Journey of Hope, or led by mental health service professionals, typically provide families with information about mental illness, emotional support, and opportunities for advocacy. Foremost, however, support groups provide a sense of community, through reciprocal exchanges of concerns, counseling, and caring, that makes members feel accepted and understood (Heller and others, 1997; Levine and Perkins, 1988).

Recent research has found that most family support group participants are Caucasian (Brady, Goldman, and Wandersman, 1994; Cox, 1993; Norton, Wandersman, and Goldman, 1993; Wood and Parham, 1990). NAMI group members, for example, are characteristically Caucasian, middle-class, and highly educated (Francell, Conn, and Gray, 1988). Similarly, a recent evaluation of Journey of Hope family support groups found that 94 percent of participants were Caucasian (Pickett, Cook, and Laris, 1997).

Several factors may underlie this trend. First, minority families—defined here as African American, Hispanic American, Asian American, and Native American families—experience greater poverty and have less formal education than Caucasian families, factors that may limit their ability to access and receive appropriate care for their ill relative and support services for themselves (Ginsberg, 1991; Kuo and Tsai, 1986; LaFramboise, 1988; McLoyd, 1990; Snowden and Cheung, 1990). Second, minority families' cultural understandings of the nature of mental illness and its causes may differ from Caucasian views. For example, Hispanic families often describe the illness as *nervios*, a term that implies emotional or somatic distress related not to the individual but to something outside him or her, such as a relationship problem. Spiritualism also is part of many Hispanics' conception of mental illness: bad spirits may cause the illness, and good spirits, or *Dios* (God), may intervene and heal the illness (Jordan, Lewellen, and Vandiver, 1995).

Third, minority families' beliefs about caregiving and the treatment and coping methods they prefer often differ from those of Caucasians. All minority groups studied have embraced a caregiving ideology that holds that ill individuals are to be cared for within the family home and that the family is obligated to provide care (Connell and Gibson, 1997; Guarnaccia and Pilar, 1996; LaFramboise, 1988; Pearson, 1992). African American families report relying on an extended network of family and friends to help them cope with their loved one's illness, as well as prayer, their pastor, and church members (Anderson, 1990; Connell and Gibson, 1997; Guarnaccia and Pilar, 1996; Wood and Parham, 1990). Urdaneta, Saldaña, and Winkler (1995) found that Mexican American families often called upon the services of a *curandero*, or folk healer, or used home remedies to treat their ill relative. Family provision of care for an ill relative is also the expected norm for Asian Americans (Pearson, 1992). However, many Asian Americans consider the disclosure of personal problems beyond the family inappropriate, something that damages the reputation and integrity of the family, and thus they may keep a relative's illness secret from extended kin and friends (Huang, 1989). Native American families may rely on traditional healing rituals that involve the ill individual, the family, and tribal members (Vraniak and Pickett, 1993).

Fourth, different levels of access to appropriate services and different attitudes toward service providers may also be factors affecting support group participation. For example, African American families often have more unmet service needs, and they tend to be suspicious of and disagree with mental health professionals about their ill relative's prognosis (Boyd-Franklin, 1989; Jordan, Lewellen, and Vandiver, 1995). Hispanic families show a greater deference to authority and have been found to be less involved in the decision to hospitalize the ill relative (Garcia-Preto, 1982; Guarnaccia and Pilar, 1996). This may be due in part to language barriers and the lack of mental health professionals who speak Spanish. Asian American families, particularly refugee families such as Laotians and Cambodians, also face language barriers, and they often do not know how to access the mental health service system (Sands, 1991; Vandiver, Jordan, Keopraseuth, and Yu, 1995). Along with this, Asian Americans often perceive severe stigma related to mental illness, resulting in feelings of shame and isolation and a reluctance to access services (Lin and others, 1982; Okazaki, 1997). Native American families report that Caucasian mental health providers often are insensitive and do not respond to their needs (LaFramboise, 1988).

Although it is possible that relatively few minority families participate in support groups because of differences in socioeconomic conditions, beliefs about mental illness, family caregiving beliefs, and access and availability of services, it is also possible that these factors affect how minority families perceive their participation in support groups. Given Levine's theory of homogenization (1988), according to which individuals whose characteristics best match the group are allowed to join, minority families may feel that they do not "fit in" with others in family support groups. They may feel that they are less accepted by and receive less support from other group members—the majority of whom are likely Caucasian. Similarly, minority families may feel uncomfortable sharing their needs, and they may be less involved in the group's activities. As a result of feeling that they do not fit in, minority families may experience lower levels of satisfaction with the group.

To date little is known about the support group experiences of minority families. The purpose of the study reported in this chapter was to explore the perceptions of minority family members regarding their support group participation. These findings may provide insight into why so few minority families attend support groups and what steps might be taken to increase their participation.

Method

Subjects. The 131 subjects who participated in the study were members of fourteen separate support groups for families of persons with mental illness. They included 104 Caucasian participants, 8 Native Americans, 7 Hispanic (non-Caucasian) participants, 6 African Americans, 4 Asian Americans, and 1 participant who self-described as "other" (non-Caucasian). Although the preferred analytic procedure is to examine each ethnic group individually (Pickett, 1995), non-Caucasian participants' data were combined, since each distinct group consisted of less than ten individuals. The sample thus consisted of 26 minority participants and 104 Caucasian participants. The underrepresentation of minorities in the sample provides anecdotal evidence of the lower use of support groups among these families.

The fourteen support groups ranged in size from four to twenty-six people, with an average of thirteen members. The groups met at least once a month and provided time for emotional support and information sharing. Ten of the groups were led by family members, and four were led by mental health service professionals. Three of the groups were composed of only Caucasian members; one group consisted of all Hispanic members; one group was predominantly African American (77 percent); and the remaining nine groups were predominantly Caucasian (77–90 percent).

Table 5.1 presents the subjects' demographic and support group participation characteristics as well as characteristics of their ill relatives. The minority and Caucasian participants were similar in terms of gender and age. Compared to the Caucasian group members, the minority participants had significantly lower levels of education (11.96 years for minorities versus 14.61 years for Caucasians), $t(126) = 3.27, p < .01$, and lower incomes (\$10,000–\$19,000 per year

Table 5.1. Demographic Characteristics of Minority and Caucasian Subjects

	Minority Subjects (n = 26)	Caucasian Subjects (n = 104)
Gender		
Male	n = 5 (19 percent)	n = 26 (25 percent)
Female	n = 21 (81 percent)	n = 78 (75 percent)
Mean age	54.87 years	56.86 years
Mean level of education	11.96 years	14.61 years
Mean annual income	$10,000–$19,000	$30,000–$39,000
Employment status		
Employed	n = 9 (35 percent)	n = 64 (62 percent)
Unemployed	n = 16 (65 percent)	n = 40 (38 percent)
Mean group tenure	25.40 months	39.34 months
Group leadership		
Professional-led	n = 12 (46 percent)	n = 24 (23 percent)
Family-led	n = 14 (54 percent)	n = 80 (77 percent)
Group composition		
White only	—	n = 13 (13 percent)
Mostly white	n = 16 (62 percent)	n = 89 (85 percent)
Mostly minority	n = 10 (38 percent)	n = 2 (2 percent)
Mean group size	8.41	10.27
Relationship to ill relative		
Parent	n = 19 (73 percent)	n = 65 (63 percent)
Sibling	n = 5 (19 percent)	n = 20 (19 percent)
Spouse	n = 2 (8 percent)	n = 5 (5 percent)
Adult child	—	n = 5 (5 percent)
Other relative	—	n = 7 (7 percent)
Friend	—	n = 1 (1 percent)
Ill relative's gender		
Male	n = 17 (65 percent)	n = 70 (68 percent)
Female	n = 9 (35 percent)	n = 33 (32 percent)
Mean age of ill relative	35.72 years	37.51 years
Mean length of illness	16.33 years	17.20 years
Mean number of days hospitalized in past six months	16.08 days	17.66 days
Diagnosis		
Schizophrenia	n = 16 (62 percent)	n = 54 (52 percent)
Other	n = 10 (38 percent)	n = 50 (48 percent)
Residential status		
Lives with subject	n = 12 (46 percent)	n = 31 (30 percent)
Does not live with subject	n = 14 (54 percent)	n = 71 (70 percent)

versus $30,000–$39,000 per year), $t(121) = 4.74$, $p < .001$. Also, a greater percentage of minorities were unemployed (65 percent versus 38 percent), $\chi^2(2, N = 130) = 6.63$, $p < .05$. Regarding support group participation, a greater percentage of minority subjects attended groups led by professionals (46 percent versus 23 percent), $\chi^2(2, N = 131) = 8.02$, $p = .01$, and groups that consisted primarily of Caucasian members (62 percent versus 38 percent), $\chi^2(4, N = 131) = 35.47$, $p < .001$. Although the Caucasian subjects appeared to have longer group tenures and attended larger groups than did the minority subjects, these differences between the two groups of subjects for these variables were not statistically significant.

The minority and Caucasian subjects were similar in terms of their ill relative's demographic and psychiatric illness characteristics. The majority of both the minority and the Caucasian subjects were parents of a person with mental illness. Most of the ill relatives were male and in their late thirties. Overall they had been ill for an average of seventeen years, and in the past six months they had spent, on average, seventeen days in a psychiatric hospital. The majority of the ill relatives had a diagnosis of schizophrenia and did not reside with the subject.

Measures. Each of the subjects completed a detailed survey that, in addition to collecting demographic information, assessed several areas related to support group participation. For the purposes of the study the following areas were examined: perceptions of group involvement and structure, and overall satisfaction with the support group.

Group involvement, structure, and satisfaction were measured by the Maton Support Group Assessment Scale (Maton, 1988). This instrument consists of five subscales measuring support provided by group members, support received from group members, friendships, role differentiation, and overall group satisfaction. Subjects were instructed to rate how accurately each item reflected their support group experience, with 1 indicating "not at all accurate" and 5 indicating "completely accurate." The items were then summed according to their respective subscale. The first subscale, *support provided* by group members to other group members, consists of four items such as "I regularly reach out and provide emotional support to group members." *Support received* by group members during meetings from other group members consists of four items such as "Members regularly reach out and provide emotional support to me." The third subscale, *friendship,* contains five items measuring friendship development between group members, such as "I have developed a close friendship with another group member." *Role differentiation,* the fourth subscale, consists of five items assessing how group tasks and duties are distributed among group members, such as "Positions of responsibility are spread among members of the group." The fifth subscale, group *satisfaction,* consists of four items and measures members' satisfaction with the support group, such as "Overall, I am very satisfied with how the group helps its members."

Analysis and Results. We conducted *t* tests to compare minority and Caucasian subjects' scores on each of the Maton subscales. As shown in Table 5.2, we found significant differences between the two groups only for friendship and overall group satisfaction. Minority subjects reported higher friendship development scores; they also reported higher levels of satisfaction with the support group.

We also conducted *t* tests to determine whether differences in friendship development and group satisfaction existed between minority subjects who attended mostly Caucasian groups and minority subjects who attended mostly

Table 5.2. Results of the *t* Tests

	Minority Subjects' Mean Score	Caucasian Subjects' Mean Score	t Value	Significance Level
Provide support	13.16	14.51	1.34	.15
Receive support	15.84	15.59	−.30	.76
Friendship	16.80	14.87	−2.22	.03
Role differentiation	16.17	16.74	.59	.56
Satisfaction	20.42	17.64	−2.56	.02

minority groups. For friendship development, the mean score for those attending mostly Caucasian groups was 16.87, compared to 16.80 for those attending mostly minority groups. This difference was not significant, $t(23) = .04$, $p = .97$. Differences between satisfaction scores also were nonsignificant (20.60 versus 19.75), $t(17) = 3.79$, $p = .73$.

Discussion

Given the small number of minority subjects, there are limitations to the findings from the study, particularly regarding specific results for each ethnic group. That is, it cannot be determined whether the findings are representative of one group (for example, do Asian Americans have the highest levels of satisfaction compared to all other subjects?) or of how each minority group differs from the others (for example, do Native Americans provide more support to group members than do Hispanics?). However, these findings do provide some insight into the outcomes of support group participation for minorities as well as suggestions for future services for these families.

The results of the study suggest that ethnic minority family support group participants develop more friendships with other group members and are more satisfied with the group itself than are Caucasian support group participants. The finding that minority subjects had more friends in their groups reflects the caregiving literature, which notes that a fundamental coping resource among minority families—particularly African Americans—is an extended network of family and friends (Anderson, 1990; Guarnaccia and Pilar, 1996). Developing and maintaining friendships with other group members may have been a natural coping response for minority subjects, that is, a bonding together with others when facing adversity. In the predominantly minority-member groups, examples of such friendships included members' sharing transportation to and from meetings and providing community meals during meetings. This higher friendship development among group members for minority subjects appears not to be an effect of attending a mostly minority group, given that the difference in friendship development scores between minority subjects who participated in mostly minority groups and those who attended mostly Caucasian groups was not significant. In other words, minority members' higher level of friendships with other group members appears not to be related to the racial homogeneity of the group.

When considered in light of the second significant finding, that minority subjects reported higher levels of satisfaction, it is easy to speculate that having more friends in one's support group may be related to greater satisfaction with the group. Yet the correlation between friendship and satisfaction for minority subjects was nonsignificant ($r = .29$, $p = .25$). However, support received and satisfaction were significantly and positively related ($r = .65$, $p < .01$), suggesting that minority subjects who received more assistance from other group members were more likely to perceive the support group as having met their needs.

As prior studies have noted, minority family members are often most in need of information about the causes of mental illness and treatments for it and face more barriers when dealing with the service system (Pickett, 1995; Urdaneta, Saldaña, and Winkler, 1995). Additional analyses (not shown) found that, compared to the Caucasian subjects, the minority subjects reported more unmet service needs, and only a small proportion were involved in advocacy activities or had read materials about mental illness. Thus the minority subjects may have had a greater need for information, which they received from other group members. Because a significantly greater percentage of the minority subjects attended groups led by professionals—presumably a more authoritative source of information and advice—this factor may also have led to greater satisfaction. The combined receipt of information and emotional support may therefore account for the minority subjects' higher levels of satisfaction with the group.

Issues of Cultural Competence

Although the minority families in the study expressed high levels of satisfaction with the support groups they attended, there is always room for improvement. The reality remains that, compared to Caucasians, few minority families of persons with mental illness participate in support groups, despite the fact that a growing number of minorities are receiving mental health care services (Cheung and Snowden, 1990). If existing support groups are to succeed in their efforts to actively involve minority families, they will need to first become culturally competent (Boyd-Franklin, Smith-Morris, and Bry, 1997). As outlined by Cook and Knox (1994), this involves identifying and understanding other cultures' values, ideologies, and beliefs and their relationship to the larger world through watching, listening to, and reading about the culture. This also means being aware of the different beliefs about mental illness and family caregiving held by minority families and understanding the coping resources they use.

In other words, cultural competence involves more than simply providing language-specific services or befriending minority families who are new to the group. Cultural competence, as it applies to support groups for families of persons with mental illness, means having an awareness of how minority families perceive and cope with mental illness and empathically applying that awareness in interactions with group members. The results of cultural *incompetence* are illustrated in the following case example:

> Mrs. C is a middle-aged Hispanic mother of a twenty-five-year-old son with paranoid schizophrenia. She has been a regular participant in a support group that consists predominantly of Caucasian families. During her turn to share her concerns, she tells the group that her son, who recently stopped taking his medication, has lost his job and returned home. He has become increasingly symptomatic, and she admits that her attempts to get him to see his psychiatrist have failed. She asks the group for advice on what to do next. One of the Caucasian mothers in the group chides her, "What is he doing living at home? Why did you let him come back? He is an adult and should be living on his own!" Several of the Caucasian group members suggest that she tell her son he cannot live at home unless he agrees to take his medication.
>
> Mrs. C is visibly appalled by this advice. "He is not in control of himself, and I cannot do this, I cannot put him out on the streets where he might get hurt. I would never ask any of my children to leave my home." A few group members try to argue that her son is in control of his behavior, since he has made the decision to stop taking his medication. Mrs. C grows quiet, and the group moves on to another member's problem. Mrs. C does not return to the group.

Had the Caucasian group members been culturally competent, they would have understood that in Hispanic families, interdependence is valued over independence (Guarnaccia and Pilar, 1996) and that it is common for children not to leave home until they marry. They also would have understood that Mrs. C may have attributed her son's illness to *nervios,* or somatic or emotional distress that is not his fault and is out of his control. Mrs. C's cultural norms dictated that her son should live at home like her other unmarried adult children, and since he was unable to control his symptoms, home was the place where he would be safe and best cared for. Had the group been culturally competent they might have refrained from promoting the Caucasian ideal of independence and instead offered her other suggestions on how to cope with her son's symptoms, such as contacting a psychiatric home visiting program.

Another factor involved in cultural competence is understanding the role primary community organizations play in involving minority families in support services (Boyd-Franklin, Aleman, Jean-Gilles, and Lewis, 1995; Boyd-Franklin, Smith-Morris, and Bry, 1997; Cook and Knox, 1993, 1994; Jordan, Lewellen, and Vandiver, 1995; Vandiver, Jordan, Keopraseuth, and Yu, 1995). One example of this is an outreach project recently initiated by an African American family support group in Chicago. Seeking a way to help other African Americans with family members suffering from mental illness, two mothers from this group, who also attended one of the largest African

Methodist Episcopal churches in the city, asked their pastor if they could participate in a church-sponsored health fair and speak about their experiences during a Sunday morning service. The pastor and church council approved the request and helped publicize the activities in the church bulletin. During the health fair, group members sat at a booth and handed out information packets on mental illness to interested individuals. Next, every Sunday for one month, members of the support group and their ill family members briefly shared with the congregation their experiences in coping with mental illness. Group members were available after the service to meet with church members who wanted more information about mental illness, about where to seek treatment, or about the support group itself. As a result of these efforts, several members of the congregation were able to access appropriate treatment for their ill relatives; others sought support for themselves by attending the group; and the pastor began to refer individuals to the support group.

In this example of cultural competence, support group members were aware of the importance of the church and church leaders in African American communities. Rather than acting on their own, group members enlisted the assistance of key church leaders (the pastor and church council). This organizational approval may have helped legitimize the group's activities in the eyes of the families they were trying to reach, and in turn it may have enabled these families to seek the services they needed for their relatives with mental illness.

Conclusion

Minority families have a great deal to teach others about coping with severe mental illness, particularly in terms of the power of sharing their burdens and of faith and hope (Lefley, 1990). For example, minority families express greater belief in an eventual cure for their ill relative, a belief not commonly shared by Caucasian families (Guarnaccia and Pilar, 1996). Incorporating alternative ways of thinking about and coping with mental illness may be beneficial for families of all ethnicities. Mental health professionals and family support group members alike need to listen to all of the voices, and greater efforts should be exerted toward understanding, appreciating, and including these differences in supportive services to families.

References

Anderson, L. P. "Acculturative Stress: A Theory of Relevance to Black Americans." *Clinical Psychology Review*, 1990, *11*, 685–702.

Boyd-Franklin, N. *Black Families in Therapy: A Multisystems Approach*. New York: Guilford Press, 1989.

Boyd-Franklin, N., Aleman, J., Jean-Gilles, M., and Lewis, S. "Cultural Competency Model: African-American, Latino and Haitian Families with Pediatric HIV/AIDS." In N. Boyd-Franklin, G. Steiner, and M. Boland (eds.), *Children, Families, and AIDS/HIV: Psychosocial and Therapeutic Issues*. New York: Guilford Press, 1995.

Boyd-Franklin, N., Smith-Morris, T., and Bry, B. H. "Parent and Family Support Groups with African American Families: The Process of Family and Community Empowerment." *Cultural Diversity and Mental Health,* 1997, *3* (2), 83–92.

Brady, C., Goldman, C., and Wandersman, A. "Similarities and Differences in Caregiver Adaptation: Focus on Mental Illness and Brain Injury." *Psychosocial Rehabilitation Journal,* 1994, *18,* 35–48.

Cheung, F. K., and Snowden, L. R. "Community Mental Health and Ethnic Minority Populations." *Community Mental Health Journal,* 1990, *26* (3), 277–291.

Connell, C. M., and Gibson, G. D. "Racial, Ethnic, and Cultural Differences in Dementia Caregiving: Review and Analysis." *The Gerontologist,* 1997, *37* (3), 355–364.

Cook, J. A., and Knox, J. "NAMI Outreach Strategies to African American and Hispanic Families: Results of a National Telephone Survey." *Innovations and Research,* 1993, *2* (3), 35–42.

Cook, J. A., and Knox, J. *Outreach to African American and Hispanic Families: A Manual for NAMI Affiliates.* Chicago: National Research and Training Center on Psychiatric Disability, 1994.

Cox, C. "Service Needs and Interests: A Comparison of African American and White Caregivers Seeking Alzheimer Assistance." *American Journal of Alzheimer's Disease,* May-June 1993, pp. 33–40.

Francell, C., Conn, V., and Gray, D. "Families' Perceptions of Burdens of Care for Chronic Mentally Ill Relatives." *Hospital and Community Psychiatry,* 1988, *39,* 1296–1300.

Garcia-Preto, N. "Puerto Rican Families." In M. McGoldrick, M. Pearce, and J. Giordano (eds.), *Ethnicity and Family Therapy.* New York: Guilford Press, 1982.

Ginsberg, E. "Access to Health Care for Hispanics." *Journal of the American Medical Association,* 1991, *261,* 238–241.

Guarnaccia, P. J., and Pilar, P. "Ethnicity, Social Status, and Families' Experiences of Caring for a Mentally Ill Family Member." *Community Mental Health Journal,* 1996, *32* (2), 243–260.

Heller, T., and others. "Benefits of Support Groups for Families of Adults with Mental Illness." *American Journal of Orthopsychiatry,* 1997, *67* (2), 187–198.

Huang, L. N. "Southeast Asian Refugee Children and Adolescents." In J. T. Gibbs, L. N. Huang, and Associates, *Children of Color: Psychological Interventions with Minority Youth.* San Francisco: Jossey-Bass, 1989.

Jordan, C., Lewellen, A., and Vandiver, V. "Psychoeducation for Minority Families: A Social Work Perspective." *International Journal of Mental Health,* 1995, *23* (4), 27–43.

Kuo, W. H., and Tsai, Y. M. "Social Networking, Hardiness, and Immigrants' Mental Health." *Journal of Health and Social Behavior,* 1986, *27,* 113–149.

LaFramboise, T. D. "American Indian Mental Health Policy." *American Psychologist,* 1988, *43,* 388–397.

Lefley, H. P. "Culture and Chronic Mental Illness." *Hospital and Community Psychiatry,* 1990, *41,* 277–286.

Levine, M. A. "An Analysis of Mutual Assistance." *American Journal of Community Psychology,* 1988, *16,* 167–188.

Levine, M. A., and Perkins, D. *Principles of Community Psychology: Perspectives and Applications.* New York: Oxford University Press, 1988.

Lin, K., and others. "Ethnicity and Family Involvement in the Treatment of Schizophrenic Patients." *Journal of Nervous and Mental Disease,* 1982, *170,* 631–633.

Maton, K. I. "Social Support, Organizational Characteristics, Psychological Well-Being, and Group Appraisal in Three Self-Help Group Populations." *American Journal of Community Psychology,* 1988, *17,* 729–753.

McLoyd, V. C. "The Impact of Economic Hardship on Black Families and Children: Psychological Distress, Parenting, and Socioemotional Development." *Child Development,* 1990, *61,* 311–346.

Norton, S., Wandersman, A., and Goldman, C. "Perceived Costs and Benefits of Member-ship in a Self-Help Group: Comparisons of Members and Non-Members of the Alliance for the Mentally Ill." *Community Mental Health Journal,* 1993, *29,* 143–160.

Okazaki, S. "Seeking Help for Schizophrenia: Asian American Patients and Their Families." Paper presented at the annual meeting of the American Psychological Association, Chicago, Aug. 18, 1997.

Pearson, V. "Community and Culture: A Chinese Model of Community Care for the Men-tally Ill." *International Journal of Social Psychiatry,* 1992, *38,* 163–178.

Pickett, S. A. "Diversity in Family Experience: Research on Ethnic Minority Families." Paper presented at the National Institute of Mental Health and Center for Mental Health Ser-vices conference "Designing Programs for Families and Consumers Based on Research on the Family Experience with Severe Mental Illness," St. Louis, Mo., Sept. 1995.

Pickett, S. A., Cook, J. A., and Laris, A. *The Journey of Hope: Final Evaluation Report.* Chicago: National Research and Training Center on Psychiatric Disability, University of Illinois at Chicago, 1997.

Sands, R. *Clinical Social Work Practice in Community Mental Health.* New York: Merrill, 1991.

Snowden, L. R., and Cheung, F. K. "Use of Inpatient Mental Health Services by Members of Ethnic Minority Groups." *American Psychologist,* 1990, *45,* 347–355.

Urdaneta, M. L., Saldaña, D. H., and Winkler, A. "Mexican-American Perceptions of Severe Mental Illness." *Human Organizations,* 1995, *54* (1), 70–76.

Vandiver, V. L., Jordan, C., Keopraseuth, K., and Yu, M. "Family Empowerment and Ser-vice Satisfaction: An Exploratory Study of Laotian Families Who Care for a Family Mem-ber with Mental Illness." *Psychiatric Rehabilitation Journal,* 1995, *19* (1), 47–54.

Vraniak, D. A., and Pickett, S. A. "Improving Interventions with American Ethnic Minority Children: Recurrent and Recalcitrant Challenges." In T. Kratochwill and R. Morris (eds.), *The Handbook of Psychotherapy with Children.* Needham Heights, Mass.: Allyn & Bacon, 1993.

Wood, J. B., and Parham, I. A. "Coping with Perceived Burden: Ethnic and Cultural Dif-ferences in Alzheimer's Family Caregiving." *Journal of Applied Gerontology,* 1990, *9,* 325–339.

SUSAN A. PICKETT is assistant professor of psychology in psychiatry at the National Research and Training Center on Psychiatric Disability, University of Illinois at Chicago.

JUDITH A. COOK is professor of sociology in psychiatry and director of the National Research and Training Center on Psychiatric Disability, University of Illinois at Chicago.

TAMAR HELLER is associate professor at the Institute on Disability and Human Devel-opment, University of Illinois at Chicago.

*Clinical issues in serving Indochinese families with a member with
severe mental illness are discussed, together with culturally relevant
strategies for engagement, communication, psychoeducational
interventions, and reinforcing natural support systems.*

Family Wisdom and Clinical Support: Culturally Relevant Practice Strategies for Working with Indochinese Families Who Care for a Relative with Mental Illness

Vikki L. Vandiver, Kham-One Keopraseuth

Over the past two decades mental health professionals have become increasingly aware of the needs of families caring for a mentally ill relative. One subset of this population that is now gaining attention as well is Indochinese families. Clinical observations suggest that Indochinese families need assistance in caring for a mentally ill relative but do not know how to access or participate in the mental health care system. Similarly, mental health professionals are often unfamiliar with the diverse languages, cultures, and health care practices of Indochinese peoples. Consequently, clinicians are having difficulty establishing an effective response to the Indochinese community. Many mental health care professionals do not have in place culturally relevant practice strategies that embrace the belief systems and traditions of Indochinese families. In addition, the stigma attached to mental illness and psychological problems is an especially difficult barrier that separates clinicians and families. Further, most studies on Indochinese refugees have tended to focus on problems, pathology, limitations, and barriers, while ignoring family knowledge and assets (Okun, 1996).

This chapter is intended as an overview for clinicians who are beginning to work with Indochinese families with a family member with mental illness. The issues and strategies it presents reflect common themes that clinicians may encounter. It is important to stress that these observations and recommendations are general ones and should be treated as guideposts rather than prescriptions. There is no typical Indochinese family, and it is not our intent to try to speak for all Indochinese groups. The chapter discusses demographic and immigration trends among Indochinese peoples; Indochinese family structures; prevalent mental disorders; clinical considerations, including gender issues, verbal and nonverbal communication, belief systems, and traditional support systems; and strategies for culturally relevant practice, including family-clinician communication, engagement and assessment, interventions, family psychoeducation, and coping. The chapter concludes by suggesting that a family-centered, community-based approach offers an effective, culturally relevant way to work with Indochinese families who have a family member with a mental illness.

Before beginning clinical work with Indochinese clients and families, clinicians can benefit from a contextual understanding of this population's demographics and of immigration and historical influences that have shaped the lives of Indochinese refugee and immigrant families.

Demographics and Immigration

The U.S. Census Bureau estimates that as of 1991 more than one million Indochinese had made their home in the United States (Van-Si, 1992), with the largest populations living in the states of California (398,200), Texas (75,100), and Washington (46,800). The term *Indochinese* refers to the people of French Indochina in Southeast Asia. Indochinese people come from Cambodia, Laos, and Vietnam. Although they come from countries in the same geopolitical region, they have significantly different customs, values, languages, and social organizations, and their level of acculturation and assimilation in the United States varies as well (Van-Si, 1992; Kim, McLeod, and Shantzis, 1992).

Cambodians. Cambodian culture can be traced back to the thirteenth century. Cambodians subscribe to the Khmer religion, known as Theravada Buddhism, which is derived from the early history and cultural traditions of India. The people of Cambodia, known as Khmer, are a racial mix of indigenous tribal people and invaders from India and Indonesia. Central values in Khmer society are harmony, balance, and avoidance of conflict. Most of the Khmer who are in the United States today arrived between 1980 and 1989, having escaped or been released from refugee camps.

Laotians. Laotian culture can be traced back to the fourteenth century. The people of Laos are greatly influenced by the Brahman Buddhist tradition, which emphasizes strong moral and spiritual ties to the living and one's ancestors. Currently more than sixty-eight ethnic groups make up the people of Laos. The major groups that have settled in the United States are the Lao (Laoloom), Hmong, Iu-Mien, Kmu, Laotheung, and Thai Dam peoples (Van-Si, 1992).

Vietnamese. Vietnamese culture is tied to Chinese culture and has a known history of four thousand years. The people of Vietnam draw much of their spiritual philosophy from Confucianism. A primary tenet of Confucianism is that the self be minimized for the good of family and society; core values are respect for elders and an emphasis on loyalty and forgiveness in any relationship. Beginning in 1975, the first wave of Vietnamese people came to the United States as refugees. In contrast, the last decade has seen an increase in legal immigrants sponsored by financially secure family members.

Many Indochinese families came to the United States as part of the refugee exodus from Southeast Asia and under the Refugee Act of 1980 (Lewis, 1994). Many had suffered torture, physical abuse, rape, illness, malnutrition, forced family separation, or forced relocation. Some of these experiences occurred in labor camps, during a period when they tried to escape, or both (Dana, 1993). The stresses of acculturation and resettlement persist for many Indochinese families.

Family Structure

In spite of significant differences between the peoples of Indochina (for example, in their religion and language), one commonality is the importance of family. Traditionally, Indochinese view themselves as members of an extended family. There is a strong emphasis on family obligations, filial piety, respect for one's parents and siblings, harmonious interpersonal relationships, interdependence, and collective responsibilities and decision making (Wong, 1985). The familial network is usually composed of a wide range of members, including grandparents, parents, children, aunts, uncles, cousins, and godparents. In terms of extended family support, Kim, Snyder, and Lai-Bitker (1996) reported that Indochinese families often provide support for the extended family by living with or near one another. Since the immigration process disrupts the indigenous support networks, many families try to create a flexible extended family by maintaining a neighborhood "comfort zone" composed of neighborhoods of family and extended kin.

Indochinese families may also be described as patriarchal, with communication and authority flowing vertically downward from the male head of the family. Both guilt and shame are used extensively as social sanctions to control the behavior of family members. From early childhood, children are indoctrinated with a sense of obligation to family and the belief that one's behavior reflects on the character of one's entire family. For example, school failure, disobedience, and juvenile delinquency are viewed as sources of great shame and embarrassment to the family (Lorenzo and Adler, 1984). Shame is also ascribed when a family member has a mental illness.

Mental Disorders Among Indochinese

Longitudinal studies of Indochinese refugees continue to reveal disproportionately high rates of psychosocial stressors and mental health problems years after their initial immigration. Psychosocial stressors common to the refugee experience are loss and grief, disrupted family relationships, social isolation, status inconsistencies, culture shock, and acculturation stresses.

Depression, high levels of distress, and post-traumatic stress disorder (PTSD) are commonly reported mental health problems (Kinzie and Manson, 1987; Mollica and others, 1987). In particular, clinical studies have found that symptoms of PTSD are very common in refugee populations (Boehnlein and Kinzie, 1995). One group that has shown particularly high prevalence rates of PTSD is survivors of the genocidal Pol Pot regime that devastated Cambodia from 1975 to 1979. Major symptoms include recurring nightmares and dreams, sudden acting or feeling as if the traumatic event were happening in the present, intense distress from exposure to symbolic or similar events, acute shame or survivor guilt, and rage at the perpetrators of the traumatic event (Kinzie and others, 1984).

Symptoms of schizophrenia are high among Indochinese clients. This condition seems exacerbated by having been isolated or separated from family and relatives for prolonged periods of time.

Generally, the attitude of Indochinese toward the mentally ill is characterized by fear, rejection, and ridicule. Families may be reluctant to admit the existence of a "crazy" family member for fear of how it will reflect on the family. Consequently, the mental health symptomatology tends to be concealed. It is often not brought to clinical attention until an acute crisis occurs in the family or the family has exhausted traditional methods of help seeking (such as shamans, fortune tellers, and Buddhist monks). By this time the patient's condition may be so deteriorated that inpatient hospitalization and long-term care are the only available alternatives. An example of the consequences of delayed treatment is illustrated by the following case described by a Laotian counselor:

> Phou is a twenty-four-year-old male. He is the second oldest of eight children and the only son. All his life he had been raised to be a king. His father was a successful boxer turned public official. His mother was a homemaker and a small business vendor in an open marketplace in Laos. They came to the United States in the late 1970s. They moved from one state to the next in search of an acceptable community with a strong Laotian culture base. In Oregon they found a well-established Buddhist temple and strong civic organizations as well as public health care services. Father and son began working in the silicon manufacturing industry. The son had set a goal of becoming an engineer and eventually running one of the companies he was working for. He enrolled in courses at the local community college. One night while cramming for a math test, he began hearing voices. He developed excruciating headaches. Not wishing to alarm his family or to appear weak, he withheld this information for several months. He eventually began to lose control, becoming agitated and isolated. He became increasingly withdrawn from family activities (for example, he ceased eating meals with the family). He eventually quit school, yet he was able to work full-time over the next year. However, his paranoia and sleep problems increased. His mother, a self-proclaimed "channel master" in the community, began to perform rituals and religious services as an attempt to rid Phou of the "problem."

Despite the mother's efforts, the thought disorder persisted. Eventually, the mother contacted a Laotian counselor at the local Indochinese psychiatric program. Over the next six months the family, patient, and counselor struggled over the issue of medication compliance. When the medication began to take effect and symptoms subsided, the family and patient decided to quit the medication. Six months later Phou was admitted to the state hospital with a diagnosis of acute psychotic episode. Upon release Phou returned to the mental health program. Discussion, education, negotiation, and compromise are continuing points with the family and patient.

Clinical Considerations

If clinicians are to respond to the needs, values, lifestyles, and expectations of Indochinese families, they must first possess a foundation of knowledge about the culture. This includes an understanding of social roles, communication patterns, beliefs, and support systems.

Family Roles and Structure. In the Indochinese culture there is a strong emphasis on family systems and the identification of specific roles and proper relationships among family members. Clinicians need to be respectful of the hierarchal nature of role relationships within the Indochinese family and the reverence attributed to ancestors, older family members, and males. Cultural traditions place ancestors, male elders, and parents at the top of the hierarchy. Therefore, if the clinician is dealing with a multigenerational Indochinese family, it is advisable to approach the grandfather first and then proceed downward (Ho, 1987).

Verbal and Nonverbal Communication. Western-trained clinicians who work with Indochinese families will benefit from understanding differences in communication styles and patterns between Western and Indochinese individuals. Chung (1992) describes some of these differences. For example, Indochinese often rely on nonverbal communication, whereas European Americans rely more on words. Indochinese may speak indirectly and make their key points at the end of a discussion, in contrast to European Americans, who communicate directly and make their key points at the beginning. Many Western psychotherapies rely on verbal communication for expression of ideas and feelings, whereas Asian cultures frequently utilize nonverbal communication to express important feelings or messages (Chung, 1992). Western clinicians must learn Indochinese cultural norms in this regard to avoid misinterpreting nonverbal messages. For example, avoidance of eye contact with persons of higher social status (such as a therapist) is a cultural norm among Indochinese. Western practitioners working with Indochinese families should not misunderstand lack of eye contact as indicative of disinterest, paranoia, lack of confidence, or lack of assertiveness.

Beliefs About Health and Illness. Meichenbaum and Turk (1987) remind us that in any society, help-seeking behaviors are influenced by cultural perceptions of illness, personal and societal beliefs, and culturally sanctioned treatment methods. Regardless of the etiology of an illness, working with people of different cultures requires understanding each culture's perspective on health and illness. Failure to do so not only thwarts appreciation of the client's wisdom and that of his or her family but also reduces the clinician's ability to understand help-seeking behaviors or the failure to seek help. Kinzie (1985) suggests that many Indochinese do not differentiate between psychological, physiological, and supernatural causes of illness. Many Indochinese families explain mental illness as a supernatural event. There is a folk tradition that views illness, particularly mental illness, as the result of having offended deities or spirits. For example, medication compliance may be impossible if the member feels guilty for offending an ancestor. The task for the clinician in such a situation would be to first explore the philosophical underpinnings of the noncompliance and then proceed with a treatment plan that incorporates the expressed belief (for example, visiting the ancestor's grave site weekly before going to the clinic for medication).

Indochinese culture also views health and illness in terms of unity between mind and body. This is unlike Western cultures, which favor a dual mind-body perspective. *Mental health* and *mental illness* may be viewed as interchangeable terms by Indochinese, with traditionally felt stigmas attached to both terms if some deficiency is implied. Kirmayer (1994) suggests that an Indochinese family may view "illness" as a manifestation of social or moral problems, cosmological forces (karma, spells, spirits, or cosmic imbalances), or a physical (organic) imbalance (such as an imbalance in body humors). Physical illness may be perceived as socially acceptable but psychological illness as disgraceful (Corin, 1994). Voicing physical complaints is often considered an acceptable way of expressing demoralization, distress, and unhappiness. Consequently, clinicians need to recognize that Indochinese are more likely to discuss physical complaints than psychological or emotional problems.

Clinicians may find that Indochinese families seem reluctant to utilize mental health or social services. In part this is because these services do not emphasize physical needs over psychological needs. Additionally, service underutilization results from language barriers, service provider mismatch, and feelings of family shame and social embarrassment. Kinzie and Manson (1987) suggest that a standard of secretiveness prevails among Indochinese about sharing emotional upset, especially for those who have been victims of rape and torture while in detainment camps. This negative cultural view of mental health problems and of help-seeking behavior promotes both denial and underutilization of available services (Yen, 1992; Kim, Snyder, and Lai-Bitker, 1996). When Indochinese do use services, they tend to use the most expensive, least specific services, such as emergency room services (White-Means, 1995).

Use of Traditional Support Systems. When mental health assistance is required, Indochinese families will often seek relief first through a number of natural or traditional support systems. These include traditional healers (for example, Buddhist monks, ritual masters, or spiritual masters such as "Phii

Pawb" and "Phii Tai"), religious leaders, and family or extended family networks (especially trusted elders). Traditional treatment recommendations might include meditation, consumption of herbal teas and plants, and "coining," which is the act of applying pressure to bruise a painful area to counter pain or disease.

In the case of a person who is distraught or depressed, a family member might encourage the ill individual to seek consultation with Buddhist monks. The "treatment" offered by the monks may take the form of a story delivered as part of a sermon based on Buddha's teaching. Given the high value Indochinese place on spiritual and social bonding among families and friends, this approach would be favorably endorsed by most families as a meaningful way of coping with the illness. However, if the spiritual or pastoral relationship with the monks and the monks' efforts did not sufficiently relieve the individual's and family's suffering, the family would likely seek more formal community resources, such as an emergency room, a primary care physician, an ethnic counselor, or (less often) a mental health clinic. Clinicians should remember the importance of traditional healers in the Indochinese community and embrace their participation in treatment plans. Clinical work with Indochinese families requires working with these traditional practitioners and facilitating contact between families and traditional helping networks.

Strategies for Culturally Relevant Practice

Acquiring effective clinical skills is a professional obligation. Learning to apply those skills successfully with different ethnic groups is an important challenge for clinicians. No Western clinician will know everything about the diverse and complex world of Indochinese populations, but an openness to learning and growing will contribute to collaborative partnerships with Indochinese families. Therefore this section delineates several key strategies for developing an informed, positive, and collaborative relationship with Indochinese family members.

Helping Families Communicate with Mental Health Professionals. For some Indochinese families, interacting with mental health professionals is one of the most difficult aspects of obtaining proper care. This is due in part to language barriers; suspicion of "government" employees and services; unfamiliarity with forms, intake procedures, and interview protocols; varying levels of literacy; fear of being blamed for the condition of their mentally ill family member; and the wish to avoid conflict. McKenzie-Pollack (1996) describes a situation in which a Khmer widow refused to return to services with a woman psychiatrist because she felt she was being "interrogated—like in the labor camps." The client was offended by the direct manner in which the mental status exam questions were delivered, but the psychiatrist had no idea the client was upset. If Indochinese clients or family members are angry or upset with a clinician, they most likely will not indicate this directly. Instead, a family member may say that they cannot return due to transportation problems.

As mentioned previously, mental illness carries a particularly severe social stigma among Indochinese, and resistance to psychiatric or mental health referrals is common. The clinician should carefully analyze the family's past and present attempts to access care and its interactions with clinicians. Much will be influenced by the family's beliefs and expectations about the mental health clinician. For example, families with an adult child with mental illness may feel embarrassed about their relative's inappropriate or disruptive behavior. The challenge for the clinician is to listen and support families while teaching them about the illness and discussing the prognosis.

Kinzie (1985) summarizes the expectations of Indochinese clients and families regarding a healer, clinician, or physician. Indochinese expect and need clinicians to understand the illness or problem, explain it in understandable terms, provide active treatment to reduce symptoms (such as psychopharmacology), offer a rapid cure, validate and confirm the sickness and sick role, and reduce family stress, fear, and guilt. To meet these expectations, the clinician should be actively involved in the diagnosis and treatment, provide access to medication when possible, provide a clear explanation of the etiology of the illness, reduce symptoms, confirm or validate the sick role, and prevent anyone from being blamed for the misfortune of mental illness.

Engaging and Assessing Clients and Families. As discussed previously, it is typical for Indochinese clients and families to have sought help through other sources long before they arrive at a mental health clinic. Indeed, they may have spent years consulting fortune tellers, taking herbal medicines, or seeking spiritual guidance. Thus a successful first meeting between clinician, client, and family—one that considers the personal family history—will determine how successful future encounters will be. Clinicians should not see earlier efforts at help seeking as ineffective but as part of a culturally competent continuum of care.

Experience has shown that when Indochinese patients are required to answer too many questions during assessment interviews, they usually drop out—as illustrated by the above example of the client who felt "interrogated." Clients and families are also wary of meeting different staff members during the intake process; direct assignment to a clinician is helpful in ensuring the client's engagement in treatment. Extended evaluations and placement on waiting lists are also inappropriate. Given the cultural and environmental situation, many Indochinese clients and families are eager to resolve their conflicts and get on with their lives. Recruitment of family support is important but must be done selectively. Since mental illness carries a stigma among Indochinese and is considered a private matter by family members, it is important to talk with family members and answer their questions. For example, obtaining approval from the head of the family before proceeding with therapy can make the difference between success and failure (Lorenzo and Adler, 1984). Familial ranking also influences the relationship between the clinician and the client or family members. For example, a Khmer (Cambodian) clinician might address a client or family member as older sister, *bong,* or younger sister, *pu'on,* depending on her social standing and age (McKenzie-Pollack, 1996).

Assessment of mental disorders without a consideration of the client's and family's national identity (for example, Laotian, Cambodian, or Vietnamese) and ethnic identity (for example, Hmong) is inappropriate and may lead to less than optimal care (Castillo, 1997). To prevent stereotyping, generalizations about Indochinese people should be used only as background in assessing a particular individual and family. Clinicians must work to ensure that cultural similarities (for example, values toward family) and other commonalities (such as common Southeast Asian heritage) do not become generalizations about individuals.

The clinician should pursue the intake and assessment interview with caution and sensitivity, concentrating initially on the client's or family's chief complaint, which is often a somatic one. The idea that someone who is not a physician should be involved in the treatment process is an alien concept for many Indochinese. Remember, the idea of confiding to someone outside the family may be embarrassing and considered a betrayal of the family. The goal at intake is to obtain the patient's cooperation and participation. To achieve these ends the clinician should be supportive yet authoritative and directive. After establishing his or her credibility, the clinician will want to cover several critical historical areas: life in the homeland (including such factors as education, socioeconomic status, experience of war), the escape process (who came, who stayed, and difficulties in escaping), life in the refugee camp (length of time there and problems), and adjustment in the United States (attitudes, problems, losses, successes).

Choosing Interventions. Depending on each client's need and family members' ability to participate in the treatment process, the treatment plan can encompass many levels of intervention. Maintenance and rehabilitation for mentally ill Indochinese involves intensive follow-up and close support for the family. This may include repeated home visits; telephone contacts; concrete services, such as filling out applications for benefits, housing, and interpreter services; and at times even arranging for burial services. Mutual aid systems, community resources (such as Buddhist temples), and the extended family are important systems among this population for problem solving and goal achievement (Chung, 1992).

Providing Family Psychoeducation and Support. Indochinese families who have a relative with a persistent mental illness often lack knowledge about mental illness and feel isolated from potential sources of help and information. Family psychoeducation is one way to offer information about mental illness and explore coping strategies. Many clinicians may be reluctant to take on the role of teacher, but treatment is facilitated when families have opportunities to learn about the illness. Although mainstream psychoeducational approaches incorporate family and patients in a structured group-learning format, Indochinese families prefer individual or private home visits by a clinician. Groups are not appropriate formats for Indochinese family members. The clinician can make home visits to bring information or offer support. The approach would still utilize psychoeducational principles (such as providing concrete information about the illness), but the material would be offered in a more private setting.

Another component of psychoeducation that needs to be modified for use with Indochinese families is the practice of lecturing on lifestyle or family behaviors. Western medicine tends to stress lifestyle changes to reduce health risks. Indochinese do not usually subscribe to such notions, nor do they respond to the direct approach used in health care education programs. The direct lecture approach may be interpreted as highlighting weakness in the individual, which would cause the family member or client to lose face, a situation that borders on shame. Instead of talking about changing lifestyles, clinicians can give directives that ultimately achieve the same outcome. For example, if excessive alcohol consumption is identified as a client and family problem, the clinician might tell the family, "For your son's best interest, I want you, as a family, to stop drinking." The clinician would then work with the family to find alternative "activities" to replace drinking behaviors and offer new skills and strategies to support the desired behavior (for example, call a friend or call the clinician). The clinician might also give each family member a "family task" or a specific job related to implementing the new strategies (a homework assignment of some sort) and ask the family to report back. This approach helps the family restructure their understanding of the problem as it changes unrealistic expectations. By incorporating the whole family into the problem solving, the power of the family stays intact.

For many mentally ill Indochinese clients and their families, adjustment in the United States is a lifelong process. The recommended approach for Indochinese clients and families dealing with cultural and social adjustment is open-ended, long-term, predictable contact using supportive and educative (psychoeducational) sessions or meetings. For example, family members would facilitate the participation of their mentally ill relative in weekly support groups. These sessions would involve topics such as medication, current events, children, financial problems, welfare reform, legal issues, employment, selecting the best health plan, and immigration and citizenship issues. Such sessions provide the added benefits of a chance for the clinician to monitor medication compliance and meaningful social supports for the family. Family members can also be of help in monitoring medication use and in encouraging continuation of programs established by the clinician.

Offering Coping Strategies. Many Indochinese clients and families have experienced multiple losses and changes in their lives, over which they have had little control. As families try to focus on coping, they may be reluctant to discuss their parallel feelings of loss. Therefore the clinician needs to initiate questions about loss and discuss the continuing balance that occurs between grieving and creative coping.

Coping strategies that are valued by the entire family should be encouraged. For Indochinese families it is important to have the entire family involved in monitoring medication compliance, scheduling checkups, and going to temple or other religious services that are a part of the family's life. In addition, clinicians working with Indochinese families with a mentally ill relative need to remind the family of how well, in fact, they are doing. Families are not usually told that they are doing well, that they are meeting the mentally ill person's needs and doing a good job adjusting to social and economic changes. The ultimate goal is to enhance the family's competence, and this can be done with direct statements, information sharing, understanding, and praise.

Using Communication Strategies in the Helping Process. Indochinese culture values harmony in general, and Indochinese may thus tend to avoid any direct conflict with clinicians, organizations, and the host community (Chung, 1992). When working with Indochinese families, therefore, any attempt to use a confrontational approach in the helping process would be counterproductive. The preferred approach is for the clinician to start with an attitude of sincerity, demonstrating an empathic, client- and family-centered outlook. One Laotian counselor shared his response to a family member who was concerned about her mentally ill nephew: "Yes, Auntie, I understand; I sympathize with your sadness. You are doing a good job at keeping Katkeo safe. Now, this is what we must do." It is also important to offer reassurance to families. One example of providing reassurance while maintaining the perception of authority is provided by the following discussion between a Laotian counselor and a Lao family whose eldest son had just been diagnosed with schizophrenia: "Mental illness exists in this world. It is not unique, and many people experience it. We know how to take care of it. Doctors are more knowledgeable. The government can help with some of the finances. Our goal is to make your load lighter. This society well tolerates people with this kind of problem. You must prepare yourself to accept the illness. Whatever your faith is, do it. If I can help connect you to resources, that is my job. We will do this together."

Taking such an active and directive approach matches family expectations of the health professional's authority and expertise (Boehnlein, 1990). In many ways the clinician acts not as a traditional therapist but as a cultural broker who can help both family members and clients understand and negotiate the challenges of acculturation and adjustment to successful daily living.

Conclusion

Three primary themes emerge when considering how best to work with Indochinese families with a mentally ill family member. First, in all likelihood the family will have already pursued a number of other, traditional interventions prior to seeing a clinician, and the clinician must recognize and support these efforts as culturally competent measures. Second, because of the strong stigma attached to mental illness in Indochinese culture, the client and family are more likely to discuss physical complaints than psychological symptoms, and this should be seen as a reflection of the Indochinese concept of mind-body integration. Third, the patient must be evaluated within the context of the family, and the clinician must support the entire family in order to help the client. In an effort to support the family, the clinician should educate family members about the health aspects of mental illness and how mental illness is a biological fact that must be addressed.

Chung (1992) reminds us that Indochinese families who care for a relative with mental illness must be understood in the context of their personal life journey and their social environment. Ultimately, mental illness is inherently unsettling for any family, and the worse the illness or disability, the more unbalancing it is. Thus clinicians should work with family members, using concrete strategies for responding to an illness episode.

In summary, working with Indochinese families requires a respectful approach that embraces family wisdom, values, and beliefs and appreciates indigenous community resources. Programs must be culturally relevant and ethnic-group-specific. Since each group and family views itself as separate and unique, treatment plans should be set up to reflect the norms, values, and language of the targeted family. Clinicians need to utilize natural support systems. For example, mutual assistance associations and local temples may be the best vehicles for managing daily support and referrals, since they have the best knowledge of community structures, family networks, and cultural issues.

Programs must provide basic social survival skills training, including training in banking, shopping, and education skills (including English language classes). Level of education is predictive of how well clients and families will be able to incorporate information on mental illness. Since a great deal of the health care and social service system is organized around the assumption of literacy in English, Indochinese families need to be equipped with language skills (Nickens, 1995).

As Indochinese families assimilate, they undergo changes in cognitive style (for example, language proficiency and preference, attitudes, knowledge of culture-specific traditions and customs, and identification preferences), values, and socioeconomic status, including changes in educational level and occupation (Marin and Van Oss Marin, 1991). Amid these significant social and cultural changes, families possess important knowledge about themselves, their mentally ill family member, and their community. Clinicians need to remember that Indochinese families are doing much more than just coping with crises; they are exploring alternative approaches to health, happiness, and stability. The clinician can be a part of that search by embracing family wisdom and extending culturally relevant clinical support services in the Indochinese community.

References

Boehnlein, J. "The Integration of Scientific Medicine with Diverse Cultural Practices." *International Journal of Mental Health*, 1990, 19 (3), 37–39.
Boehnlein, J., and Kinzie, J. "Refugee Trauma." *Transcultural Psychiatric Research Review*, 1995, 32, 223–252.

Castillo, R. *Culture and Mental Illness*. Pacific Grove, Calif.: Brooks/Cole, 1997.

Chung, D. "Asian Cultural Commonalities: A Comparison with Mainstream American Culture." In S. Furuto and others (eds.), *Social Work Practice with Asian Americans*. Thousand Oaks, Calif.: Sage, 1992.

Corin, E. "The Social and Cultural Matrix of Health and Disease." In R. Evans, M. Barer, and T. Marmor (eds.), *Why Are Some People Healthy and Others Not?* Hawthorne, N.Y.: Aldine de Gruyter, 1994.

Dana, R. H. *Multicultural Assessment Perspectives for Professional Psychology*. Needham Heights, Mass.: Allyn & Bacon, 1993.

Ho, M. *Family Therapy and Ethnic Families*. Thousand Oaks, Calif.: Sage, 1987.

Kim, S., McLeod, J., and Shantzis, C. "Cultural Competence for Evaluators Working with Asian-American Communities: Some Practical Considerations." In M. A. Orlandi (ed.), *Cultural Competence for Evaluators: A Guide for Alcohol and Other Drug Prevention Practitioners Working with Ethnic/Racial Communities*. Rockville, Md.: Office of Substance Abuse Prevention, U.S. Department of Health and Human Services, 1992.

Kim, Y., Snyder, B. O., and Lai-Bitker, A. "Culturally Responsive Psychiatric Case Management with Southeast Asians." In P. Manoleas (ed.), *The Cross-Cultural Practice of Clinical Case Management in Mental Health*. Binghamton, N.Y.: Hayworth Press, 1996.

Kinzie, J. "Overview of Clinical Issues in the Treatment of Southeast Asian Refugees." In T. Owan (ed.), *Southeast Asian Mental Health*. Washington, D.C.: National Institute of Mental Health, 1985.

Kinzie, J., and Manson, S. "The Use of Cross-Cultural Rating Scales in Cross-Cultural Psychiatry." *Hospital and Community Psychiatry*, 1987, *38* (2), 190–196.

Kinzie, J., and others. "Posttraumatic Stress Disorder Among Survivors of Cambodian Concentration Camps." *American Journal of Psychiatry*, 1984, *141*, 645–650.

Kirmayer, L. "Is the Concept of Mental Disorder Culturally Relevant?" In S. Kirk, *Controversial Issues in Mental Health*. Needham Heights, Mass.: Allyn & Bacon, 1994.

Lewis, J. "Southeast Asians in the United States." *A Profile of the Cambodian, Laotian and Vietnamese People in the United States*. Chicago: National Association for Education and Advancement, Chicago Urban League, March 1994.

Lorenzo, M., and Adler, D. "Mental Health Services for Chinese in a Community Health Center." *Social Casework*, 1984, *65*, 600–609.

Marin, G., and Van Oss Marin, B. *Research with Hispanic Populations*. Thousand Oaks, Calif.: Sage, 1991.

McKenzie-Pollack, L. "Cambodian Families." In M. McGoldrick, J. Giordano, and J. Pearce (eds.), *Ethnicity and Family Therapy*. New York: Guilford Press, 1996.

Meichenbaum, D., and Turk, D. *Facilitating Treatment Adherence: A Practitioner's Guidebook*. New York: Plenum, 1987.

Mollica, R., and others. "Indochinese Versions of the Hopkins Symptom Checklist-25: A Screening Instrument for the Psychiatric Care of Refugees." *American Journal of Psychiatry*, 1987, *144* (4), 497–500.

Nickens, H. "The Role of Race/Ethnicity and Social Class in Minority Health Status." *Health Services Research*, 1995, *30*, 151–162.

Okun, B. *Understanding Diverse Families: What Practitioners Need To Know*. New York: Guilford Press, 1996.

Van-Si, C. *Understanding Southeast Asian Cultures*. Bend, Ore.: Maverick Publications, 1992.

White-Means, S. "Conceptualizing Race in Economic Models of Medical Utilization: A Case Study of Community-Based Elders and the Emergency Room." *Health Services Research*, 1995, *30* (1), 207–223.

Wong, H. "Training for Mental Health Service Providers to Southeast Asian Refugees: Models, Strategies, and Curricula." In T. C. Owan (ed.), *Southeast Asian Mental Health: Treatment, Prevention, Services, Training and Research*. Washington, D.C.: National Institute of Mental Health, 1985.

Yen, S. "Cultural Competence for Evaluators Working with Asian/Pacific Island-American Communities: Some Common Themes and Important Implications." In M. A. Orlandi (ed.), *Cultural Competence for Evaluators: A Guide for Alcohol and Other Drug Prevention Practitioners Working with Ethnic/Racial Communities.* Rockville, Md.: Office of Substance Abuse Prevention, U.S. Department of Health and Human Services, 1992.

VIKKI L. VANDIVER is assistant professor, Graduate School of Social Work, Portland State University.

KHAM-ONE KEOPRASEUTH is senior mental health counselor and research associate, Indochinese psychiatric program, Department of Psychiatry, Oregon Health Sciences University, Portland.

Family education is a respectful approach to working with Native American families. When clinicians are informed about tribal ways, families can contribute greatly to accurate diagnosis and effective treatment and rehabilitation.

Working with Native American Families

Carmen A. Johnson, Dale L. Johnson

This chapter discusses the large number of Indian people who live in or near the Indian nations, each individually governed by sovereign tribal governments. Some reservations are essentially closed religious communities. Others readily incorporate attractive cultural items from outside the community. Successful health programs for these populations are often those that take an educational approach, because this accords respect for the people and their ways.

When working with American Indian families, a starting point is to know about the tribe and its relationships with other tribes in the area. Because the Navajo and Hopi live as neighbors does not mean that they share cultural traditions or a common language or even that they are in agreement over land boundaries. They differ in many ways. The clinician should use library resources to gain broad background information. Careful listening and sensitive questioning can provide necessary information for specific families. Attneave (1982) has cautioned against being influenced by "movies, a vacation trip, or an interest in silver jewelry. These are among the most offensive, commonly made errors when non-Indians first encounter an American Indian person or family" (p. 57).

Although, in general, families of people with serious mental illness have been neglected by mental health professionals, it seems likely that American Indian families have been neglected even more. There has been reluctance by professionals to acknowledge that serious mental illness is a problem for Indian families; emphasis has been placed on alcohol and drug problems instead, and Indian people have had to cope with the problems of serious mental illness on their own. Many Indian families live in isolated rural areas, must cope with conflicting mental health provider authorities, and put up with the lack of understanding of Indian cultures by professionals. These factors also contribute to neglect of this population.

Three important advances have occurred in psychiatry that show great promise for Native Americans. The first is the development of more meaningful diagnostic systems; at this point in time we can have as much confidence in a diagnosis of schizophrenia or affective disorder as we can in a diagnosis of cancer or heart disease. The second is the availability of effective medications that lack the undesirable side effects of earlier drugs and offer improved control of symptoms. The third is the development of effective rehabilitation methods; we now know that persons who suffer from serious mental illness need not remain gravely handicapped by their illness for life.

Where Culture Makes a Difference

Cultural differences affect the clinical management of serious mental illness, the presentation of symptoms, the lifetime course of the illness, and rehabilitation goals and methods.

Indian people, like all other people, report their experience of mental illness using the terms and concepts that are meaningful to them. Few have encountered the psychiatric terminology of Western medicine. Instead, Indian people have a rich cultural universe composed of sacred beings, spiritual concepts, interpersonal obligations and privileges, and an oral and written history apart from that of non-Indians. Elements of Indian culture (kinship obligations and privileges, for example) may be mistranslated into psychodynamic terms by an ethnocentric non-Indian clinician who believes that his or her own kinship customs are universal. Some non-Indian clinicians suspend clinical judgment as they become more and more fascinated by the imagery presented by some Indian clients. When communication with the family is difficult, an impatient or uninterested non-Indian clinician may simply neglect to get a relevant history. Most Indian families have lived together for centuries and can remember stories of relatives from other generations who experienced similar problems. These family stories can provide strong clues for the diagnosis of the client if the condition has a genetic basis, as in bipolar disorder.

Some non-Indian clinicians have concluded that diagnosable mental illness does not exist among Indian people. We have been told that certain Indian communities do not have schizophrenia, that certain others do not have bipolar disorder. We have also been told that in certain Indian communities the majority of the people have mental illness. And frequently we were told that alcoholism was the effective cause of mental illness in Indian populations.

The Native American Family Project, sponsored by the Center for Mental Health Services (CMHS), offered some quite revealing information in this regard. After hearing from white mental health workers that a particular Indian community had no bipolar disorder, because this was considered a "white man's disease," we in the project invited Indian people to sit with us in the evening and talk about mental illness. We heard the following story: "I used to be a successful businessman in [a nearby city], but I ruined it all by thinking so big and getting so wild. I turned to drinking, lost my wife and children. Finally I got so far down there was nowhere for me but to come back to the reservation. When I first got here it was spring, and the river was really rushing in the thaw. I was so high [manic] I remember telling myself that of course I couldn't walk over it, even though it looked to me as if I could. But I thought if I walked fast enough I could get across by walking on the bottom."

Fortunately for this intelligent and talented man, an alert Indian mental health worker recognized bipolar disorder and started him on the road to recovery.

In other communities we heard these examples:

"He said he could hear the heavy tread of the gods behind him everywhere he went. He used to run off into the fields, and his family would go after him and bring him back. He'd be yelling and struggling, saying that the dancers were coming for him."

"He walked barefoot through the snow all the way to the hospital."

"She set fire to their trailer house."

"We knew when he began to hurt the sheep that another spell was coming on."

"After crying all night, he drove his car into the river."

In the months to come we heard many such stories, enough to convince us that a careful diagnostic review was indicated in each of these instances, and many more. Alcoholism was not an adequate explanation. Some of the cases described involved serious mental illness, and it became clear that no community was immune to the devastation such illness brought.

One of the most serious consequences of neglecting an accurate diagnosis for Indian people is that appropriate medication cannot be initiated, and therefore the mental illness gets worse. Another problem is that the move to privatization of public health has spawned a number of health care programs that provide alternative treatments, among which Native American sweat baths and other rituals are popular. We must remember that profits are the goal of these privatization efforts. By contrast, Native American treatments are exclusively for Native Americans, as they are part of a closed religious system. Treatments for mental illness are integrated within a complex of sacred beliefs and symbols belonging only to the tribe. The removal of a specific treatment to sell to "paying customers" cheapens rather than respects the ways of Native Americans. Indian treatments, like other religious practices, should be encouraged whenever the family and individual can find comfort in them, but they should be carefully protected from prying eyes or the judgment of outsiders. A situation could develop where white people receive effective treatment for mental illness but Indian people receive, for example, sweat baths and nothing more. This type of mental health care must certainly be rejected.

Lifetime Course

Longitudinal studies (Warner, 1985) reveal an onset for schizophrenia in late adolescence or young adulthood, characterized by extremely disturbed psychotic episodes separated by short periods of respite. As the person ages, generally after thirty years of age, the periods of psychosis tend to become less severe, and the periods of respite become longer. However, residual disabilities become evident, which can only be mitigated by a concerted rehabilitation effort. Most evident are symptoms such as difficulty in self-starting, extreme sensitivity to stimulation, and short attention span.

This situation is probably the same in Indian communities, with the added problem of comorbid drug and alcohol abuse. A high prevalence of drugs and alcohol in some Indian communities may increase the severity of symptoms and complicate rehabilitation.

Treatment and Rehabilitation Goals and Opportunities

American Indian families typically view involvement of the family in the treatment process as quite natural. Indian families go to mental health professionals for help, and they are willing to support the treatment process. To do this they need information. This should be provided honestly, clearly, and directly, with ample opportunity for questions. A single information session is rarely enough. Family education, in groups, appeared to be effective during the CMHS Native American Family Project.

Families should also be referred to local affiliates of the National Alliance for the Mentally Ill (NAMI). These affiliates include Indian families, who may be able to provide information in a way that is most meaningful and acceptable to the family. Participants in the Native American Family Project found NAMI's written materials helpful. In addition, supportive family counseling as developed by Bernheim (1982) appears to be appropriate for American Indian families.

Guidelines for the treatment of schizophrenia (American Psychiatric Association, 1996), bipolar disorder (American Psychiatric Association, 1994), and depression (Depression Guideline Panel, 1993a, 1993b) are now available. These have broad applicability, and there seems to be no reason why they should not be used in treating Indian patients.

Two important bodies of literature provide some clues as to how Indian families can help their mentally ill family member, even without medication or mental health programs. The first of these is the evidence from the World Health Organization (WHO) schizophrenia study (1979). These results show that none of the nations studied were free of schizophrenia. Therefore, it is highly unlikely that an Indian community can be found in which there is no schizophrenia. Interestingly, people in the underdeveloped countries showed a somewhat later onset for schizophrenia and a more benign course than people in the industrialized nations. Nations such as India cannot hope to provide medication to all those who suffer from schizophrenia, so the more benign course shown in the WHO studies cannot be attributed to superior chemotherapy regimens. The expressed emotion (EE) studies (Koenigsberg and Handley, 1986) help to explain at least part of the observed differences between nations. In this large body of EE literature, families in underdeveloped nations, such as India, were shown to interact with their family member with mental illness with less criticism and overinvolvement than families in industrialized nations. This calmer style has been shown to be more comfortable and less likely to overstimulate a person who is highly vulnerable to stress. From these and other important sources a rehabilitation program can be devised for Native American families that can reduce stress in the environment, avoid emotional overinvolvement, increase constructive behavior, and decrease distorted thinking. The outlines of this program are presented briefly in the following pages.

Crisis Programs. Even with the buffering of medications, periodic recurrence of psychotic episodes is to be expected in cases of serious mental illness. Families need to know that if they can comfort their family member and keep him or her safe, the episode will probably resolve itself in five to ten days. The ill family member should go to a quiet place for that period of time. Some Indian people feel better inside, and some people feel better outside. Contrary to hospital practices, they may not feel better in a room alone.

When participants in the Native American Family Project discussed this matter with Indian people, an Indian physician said that the safest place he could imagine was when, as a child, he slept every night between his grandparents, with his grandfather's arm around his shoulders and his grandfather's hand on his chest, gently beating a rhythm to a soft chant. He said he couldn't imagine a solitary room being a place of comfort when he was frightened or anxious.

In any case, the family should make every effort to eliminate noise, confusion, strangers, and face-to-face demands until the sufferer feels more able to cope. Periods of acute disturbance are definitely not the time to take the person to a powwow, fiesta, shopping mall, or family reunion. Someone whom the person with mental illness trusts should remain with him or her until the episode passes.

As the disturbing symptoms abate the person will exhibit fatigue, and he or she should be allowed to sleep as long as needed, with such gentle forays into family life only as far as can be tolerated. If symptoms reappear, the family should drop back to the most sheltered care again, until such time as the sufferer announces that he or she is feeling better.

From this description of the general rules of family management of acute episodes, it can be seen that a person suffering such episodes is vulnerable to stimulation and stress. Therefore, a good strategy when an acute episode occurs is to try to think through what might have precipitated the episode, so that steps can be taken to avoid the cause in the future. Consider if an acquaintance had been to visit with alcohol or drugs to share, if a ceremonial experience was too intense, if the sufferer had watched a disturbing television program, if a trip to town was too exciting, or if a relationship was too emotional. To some extent the person with mental illness can help in this exercise, as long as it does not become blaming or threatening.

If helpful treatment is available, the time to use it is when the person is experiencing prodromal symptoms. Contact the psychiatrist. A temporary increase in medication may help at this time. The person should get more rest and reduce stress as much as possible. Once the family and the person with mental illness become accustomed to the shifts and changes of the illness, crises can often be minimized.

Remission. During periods of remission, when the family member is feeling good, it is time to become involved in rehabilitation. Physical fitness should be addressed slowly and gently. Friendly coaching in communication and social skills can be part of the family program, since these skills can be compromised severely by the illness. Crafts, animal care, farm work, or religious duties might be taken up for an hour or two a day. Usually people with mental illness feel more comfortable if they can perform their tasks out of the public eye, for short periods of time and with praise for accomplishments, however small. Possibly the person can be helped to make a friend who is willing to take time to visit for a short time every day. Lingering over coffee at a Dairy Queen can be a major social event for someone recovering from the severe insult of mental illness. Families must be reminded to go slowly in any new endeavor, allowing weeks for the person to settle into the new routine. The strain of any change may cause considerable fatigue, and extra hours of sleep may be needed.

Praise does not come naturally to many Indian families. However, a person recovering from mental illness seems to need more than the usual amount of reassurance and affection. Virtually all families that practice open and lavish praise and support for the sufferer find that it is rewarded with better feelings and performance.

One of the advantages of family management over urban or hospital rehabilitation programs is that people with mental illness find it difficult to transfer learning from one setting to a very different tribal setting. If Indian families can find a niche in the family and community for their member with mental illness, he or she will probably be able to maintain the comforting daily routine for most of his or her young adulthood, until the psychotic episodes begin to fade with age.

Indian people with serious mental illness are entitled to Supplemental Security Income (SSI) and Medicaid by virtue of their dual citizenship in their own Indian nation and in the state in which they live. Although these grants can be difficult to obtain and are usually small, they often constitute a significant portion of the income of the whole family. This can ease the burden of caring for a person with a disability, a burden that necessitates seeking help from a large extended kinship network and years of sustained effort to achieve a successful recovery. Some white social workers misunderstand Indian economic obligations and insist that SSI grants be used exclusively by and for the person with mental illness. But the "give-away" Indian economy, at one time quite common throughout Indian country, circulates goods and services by giving them away rather than getting them. This traditional economy still influences interpersonal obligations and privileges in Indian communities and should be encouraged rather than disparaged, since it strengthens the social network that supports the mentally ill person.

A Forward Glance

If rehabilitation programs were to be organized in Indian communities, the tribally controlled community colleges could offer a certificate program for mental health aides to provide a trained workforce for Indian and non-Indian communities. More and more Indian communities are becoming alcohol and drug free under the control of tribal authorities, and this is an important advantage over many non-Indian communities. The stable households and quiet, clean atmosphere can greatly support the path to recovery.

A Note About the Authors

A disclaimer: neither of us is Native American. As one Indian mother said about her son in school, "He can learn to act like a white person, but they can't teach him how to think like a white person." Likewise, we will never be Indian people. We can only hope to learn respect for the ways of people of whom we have become very fond. We find that we move easily across cultural boundaries, and seeing things from another point of view is an exhilarating experience. For that we thank the many Indian families who have befriended us over the years: We will never forget you and hope to be alert to opportunities to support the well-being of your people with serious mental illness and their courageous and loyal families whenever that becomes possible.

In the last few years Carmen has collaborated in mental health projects in the Chippewa, Dakota, and Lakota areas of North and South Dakota; among the northern Pueblos and Navajos of New Mexico, the Pima and Papago of Arizona, and the Shoshone Bannock of Utah; and in the urban Indian projects in Alaska. These projects were funded for three years by the federal Center for Mental Health Services in an effort to bring the family movement in mental illness to Indian communities. But these were only the most recent of our experiences in Indian country.

Many years ago we were privileged to work on a National Institute of Mental Health project under the direction of Dr. Bert Kaplan. This project asked what mental illness might look like in non-Western Native American cultures. Dale studied problems of mental illness with Navajo persons (Kaplan and Johnson, 1974), and Carmen did the same with Zuni people (Acosta, 1969). We both studied and consulted with Makah people on the Northwest coast and Dakota Sioux on the same project (Johnson and Johnson, 1965). Possibly the one skill that we brought to those early years in Indian country was that of clinical observation, coupled with the privilege, under the conditions of our study grant, of suspending judgment. We had the luxury of time to learn how to see problems of mental illness through Indian eyes. We were not required to determine cause, and we did not have to determine a treatment plan. Best of all, we could wait until our kindly hosts could help us understand the nature of mental illness in their own way and on their own terms.

Another matter of catastrophic proportions has occurred since our early years in Indian country, one that has made a major difference in our perception of mental illness in Indian communities. Our own son became psychotic with schizophrenia, and we have ourselves experienced for more than twenty years the chaos, violence, sorrow, and suffering that accompany untreated and poorly treated serious mental illness. This experience has made it easy for us to recognize the same story of decades of burden for Indian families whose loved ones suffer from serious mental illness.

References

Acosta, C. "Zuni Healing Societies: The Clown Fraternity." In R. Almond (ed.), *The Healing Community*. Northvale, N.J.: Aronson, 1969.

American Psychiatric Association. "Practice Guideline for the Treatment of Patients with Bipolar Disorder." *American Journal of Psychiatry,* 1994, *151* (suppl.), 1–36.

American Psychiatric Association. "Practice Guideline for the Treatment of Patients with Bipolar Disorder." *American Journal of Psychiatry,* 1996, *153* (suppl.).

Attneave, C. "American Indians and Alaska Native Families: Emigrants in Their Own Homeland." In M. McGoldrick, J. K. Pearce, and J. Giordano (eds.), *Ethnicity and Family Therapy*. New York: Guilford Press, 1982.

Bernheim, K. F. "Supportive Family Counseling." *Schizophrenia Bulletin,* 1982, *8,* 634–641.

Depression Guideline Panel. *Depression in Primary Care*. Vol. 1: *Detection and Diagnosis*. Clinical Practice Guideline no. 5 (AHCPR Publication No. 93–0550). Rockville, Md.: Agency for Health Care Policy and Research, Public Health Service, U. S. Department of Health and Human Services, 1993a.

Depression Guideline Panel. *Depression in Primary Care*. Vol. 2: *Treatment of Major Depression*. Clinical Practice Guideline no. 5 (AHCPR Publication No. 93–0550). Rockville, Md.: Agency for Health Care Policy and Research, Public Health Service, U. S. Department of Health and Human Services, 1993b.

Johnson, D. L., and Johnson, C. A. "Totally Discouraged: A Depressive Syndrome of the Dakota Sioux." *Transcultural Research Review,* 1965, *2,* 141–143.

Kaplan, B., and Johnson, D. L. "The Social Meaning of Navaho Psychopathology and Psychotherapy." In A. Kiev (ed.), *Magic, Faith and Healing: Studies in Primitive Psychiatry Today*. New York: Free Press, 1974.

Koenigsberg, H. W., and Handley, R. "Expressed Emotion: From Predictive Index to Clinical Construct." *American Journal of Psychiatry,* 1986, *143,* 1361–1373.

Warner, R. *Recovery from Schizophrenia: Psychiatry and Political Economy*. New York: Routledge, 1985.

World Health Organization. *Schizophrenia: An International Follow-up Study*. New York: Wiley, 1979.

CARMEN A. JOHNSON *is professor emeritus of health administration at Southwest Texas State University.*

DALE L. JOHNSON *is professor of psychology at the University of Houston.*

Cross-cultural studies of families' experience of mental illness are discussed, in terms of uniformities in and differences between belief systems and values, caregiving norms, perceived burden and distress, and expectations, with suggestions for further research and applications to practice.

The Family Experience in Cultural Context: Implications for Further Research and Practice

Harriet P. Lefley

Europeans, Australians, and many others use the term *carers* when referring to families of persons with mental illness. *Carers* seems to me a better term for the persons whom we in the United States typically refer to as *caregivers* or *caretakers*. The latter are functional words, anchored to tasks rather than to emotional investment. Carers are individuals who are profoundly involved with the welfare of patients or consumers, with whom their lives and happiness are most intimately entwined.

Various chapters in this issue of *New Directions for Mental Health Services* have traced the history of the relationships between clinicians and families within the context of what is essentially the Western psychodynamic paradigm. This paradigm was traditionally based on a number of premises: that defective parenting is the primary etiological antecedent of mental disorders; that individuation is a primary goal of treatment, requiring the patient's psychological separation from the family of origin; and that the therapeutic alliance is based on a level of confidentiality that precludes any communication between therapists and the patient's family members.

Although the family theories of the 1950s and 1960s subsequently delivered a different paradigm, linking symptomatology to dysfunctional family systems, in no case was the family viewed in the light of "carers." After speaking at a conference on mental illness in Western culture, I was approached by a very warm and thoughtful colleague who informed me that some words I had used had abruptly changed her mind-set. "I never thought about patients as the family's 'loved ones,' and then I suddenly realized that we're talking about these people's children, their spouses and siblings, and through it all, of course, they love them and care what happens to them." Family love is not a concept that has any currency in the clinical literature, but its reality is very much linked to patients' progress.

In the literature on transcultural psychiatry it has been evident for many years that families are viewed and treated differently in other cultures. *Loved ones* may be a Western term, but the concept of mutual caring and responsibility is implicit in family relationships. Furthermore, the notion that the patient is somehow separate from the family, that patients should be treated apart from their support systems, appears to be alien to traditional cultures. There seem to be very different concepts of self and personhood in those cultures described by social scientists as individualistic (cultures that emphasize individual boundaries and rights) versus cultures that are sociocentric or collectivist (societies that are family- and group-oriented; Triandis, 1995).

Family Roles in Individualistic and Sociocentric Cultures

Modern industrial societies tend to be individualistic, whereas more traditional cultures tend to be sociocentric or collectivist—a dichotomy that is correlated with divergent notions about independence and interdependence, with kinship structure and role obligations to persons designated as kin. Research indicates that persons in individualistic cultures have an interpersonal moral code that stresses freedom of choice and personal responsibility, whereas persons in sociocentric cultures have a duty-based interpersonal moral code that emphasizes mandatory responsibilities to others (Miller, 1994). These codes inform families' beliefs about their obligation to care for disabled relatives and the reciprocal obligation of the disabled individual to accept this caregiving as a natural right. Although the person may regret being a financial burden, being cared for by the family in itself poses no insult to one's self-worth.

In individualistic cultures, a disabled person's acceptance of family support may be psychodynamically troublesome, since it implies a posture of dependency, a reliance on others rather than oneself. Accepting help from others may be perceived as a form of weakness and an infringement on one's autonomy. In sociocentric cultures, a shared view of reciprocal obligation makes it easier for individuals to concede impairment and accept help from those whose role decrees that they provide it. Thus when illness or disability occurs, both the affected persons and their healers expect the family to be involved in all aspects of the process of diagnosis, treatment, and rehabilitation.

In traditional cultures the family is very much part of the healing process, whether through active participation or implicit support. Thus in psychiatric interventions, families typically accompany patients, are privy to the diagnosis, and are viewed as partners in therapy. In India, psychiatrists Shankar and Menon (1991) point out that families have always been viewed as allies and collaborators and that "the ideological see-saw from viewing families as schizophrenogenic in the 1950s to viewing families as equal treatment partners in the 1980s has not taken place in India" (p. 86).

Even in adaptations of psychoanalysis for non-Western patients, families are involved in treatment. Consider the contemporary ethnopsychoanalytic therapy developed by Tobie Nathan and now widely used in France with migrant patients from traditional cultures: "At the beginning of the session, the professional in charge of the patient (or the patient's representative) and the members of the patient's family are invited to present their version of the patient's problem. . . . At the end of the session . . . the patient is given a prescription, i.e., he is asked to do something that helps restore the contact with family members" (Streit, 1997, p. 333).

Other cultural psychiatrists point out that "notions regarding *confidentiality* differ across cultures. In some settings patients assume that any information conveyed to the clinician is a private and individual matter. Indeed, the laws and state apparatus may reinforce this belief. . . . In other societies the standard may be quite different. It may be assumed that anything conveyed to a clinician might be shared with the family, clan leaders, or elders. In such settings, the unit of confidentiality might be the family rather than the individual" (Westermeyer and Janca, 1997, p. 302, original emphasis).

Among immigrant groups adapting to Western culture, families are viewed as a natural support system. For example, in treating Asian American patients for major anxiety disorders, Iwamasa (1997) notes that "family members, community or religious leaders, or family friends can be used as allies in the development and implementation of interventions outside of therapy. This automatically builds in a social support component which will increase the likelihood of maintaining any gains made during treatment" (p. 123).

The availability of social support systems is, of course, a central component of the treatment of major psychiatric disorders. From a longitudinal perspective, it seems as if our clinicians in modern industrial societies are just now catching up with the wisdom long inherent in the structure of traditional cultures. Persons with severe and persistent mental illness need the support of others, and the more this can come from kinship networks—those who are related by ties of blood and mutual caring—the more the person is assured of continuity of support.

Culture and Expressed Emotion

The expressed emotion (EE) research is of particular interest in cross-cultural comparisons. There is considerable evidence that despite transcultural concordance in the predictive value of high EE, there are highly significant cultural differences in the ratios of high to low EE. Low EE seems to be normative in traditional cultures, including traditional ethnic groups in Great Britain and the United States (Jenkins and Karno, 1992). An overview of the research suggests that it is primarily among urban families of Anglo-Saxon cultural heritage (American, English, and Australian) that the number of high-EE relatives has exceeded that of low-EE relatives (Lefley, 1992). Leff (1988) has linked low EE to the better prognosis for schizophrenia in developing countries, suggesting that the extended family offers a buffering mechanism in the availability of many people to interact with and support the patient. This contrasts with the great caregiving strain imposed on the nuclear families of the West, evident in the family burden research (Lefley, 1996).

Several researchers have begun to study the attributions of high- and low-EE families and their effects on patients. Attributions underlying the hostile criticism of high-EE relatives typically have been interpreted as holding the person accountable for the symptoms and behaviors of the illness (Hooley, 1987). If a relative makes unfulfillable demands based on this premise, one can see how these attributions can make the patient decompensate. Indeed, a British study found that when family psychoeducation decreased relatives' attributional beliefs that their ill family member should be able to control their symptoms, there were commensurate reductions in hostility (Brewin, 1994).

Yet the high-EE picture is more complex than that. Another study of British families also found that highly critical relatives saw the illness as controllable by the patient (Barrowclough, Johnston, and Tarrier, 1994). Yet the other component of high EE, emotional overinvolvement, was associated with attributions of noncontrollability, similar to those of low-EE relatives. Another study by these researchers found that high EE in the family was associated with high depression scores and self-blaming attributions in relatives (Barrowclough, Johnston, and Tarrier, 1995). It seems as if attributions of personal guilt are associated with emotional overinvolvement, and attributions of client accountability are associated with hostile criticism, and both may lead to similarly negative results.

It is of great interest that these attribution studies were conducted in modern, individualistic cultures, where internal locus of control and personal responsibility are strong features of our value system. In traditional cultures external locus of control may be part of the reason for lower EE in families. However, even in the developing countries, tolerant attributions may be affected by social change and by the economic impact of mental illness on village life (Martyns-Yellowe, 1992).

Ethnic Group Differences in the United States

In cross-ethnic research on families of persons with psychiatric disabilities in the United States, racial and ethnic differences have been found in the areas of causal attribution, prognostic expectations, home caregiving, kinship roles of primary caregivers, hospitalization patterns, service utilization patterns, perceived family burden, and psychological distress. In a study of African American, Hispanic, and European American families, Milstein, Guarnaccia, and Midlarsky (1995) found that Hispanics were more likely to perceive their relatives' problems as emotional, whereas the other groups preferred a medical explanation. European Americans were more skeptical than the comparison groups about the possibility of obtaining a cure and were significantly less likely to have their relatives live at home. In Chapter Four Peter Guarnaccia indicates that in this study sample, about one-third of European American patients lived with their relatives, in contrast to three-quarters of Hispanic and 60 percent of African American patients. African American clients were the most involved in day programs; European American clients made the most use of residential services; Hispanic families did not use residential programs at all and used day treatment the least of the three ethnic groups.

Guarnaccia's study revealed that minority families tended to have larger social networks than white Americans, and these networks included more kin (Chapter Four; Guarnaccia and Parra, 1996). The African Americans and Hispanics in his study sought out other family members for advice, whereas the whites turned more to mental health professionals. White respondents reported greater effects on their physical and mental health from their caregiving role, a finding the authors attributed to lack of social support networks.

Social Networks, Kinship Roles, and Family Burden

Almost all cross-ethnic comparisons have found lower perceived burden among African American families of persons with psychiatric disabilities than among white American families (for example, Horwitz and Reinhard, 1995; Pickett, Vraniak, Cook, and Cohler, 1993; Pruchno, Patrick, and Burant, 1997; Steuve, Vine, and Streuning, 1997). Researchers have generally attributed these findings to the larger social networks among blacks and to a cultural mutual aid system that values reciprocity and social responsibility (Pruchno, Patrick, and Burant, 1997). Yet in the study by Pickett, Vraniak, Cook, and Cohler (1993), size of social networks was not necessarily related to social support. They found that black parents of severely mentally ill adults were significantly higher than white parents in coping mastery and self-esteem, but surprisingly these personality variables were negatively related to their greater number of social supports, including church resources.

The researchers felt that potential supportive resources may sometimes have an adverse effect. More extended family or a larger pool of church members who do not understand mental illness may bring additional problems. Pickett and colleagues found that African American families were disappointed by the amount of help offered by other kin. Similar findings were reported by Biegel, Milligan, and Putnam (1991). Black caregivers stated that their family members provided significantly less support than that reported by white caregivers. Yet in all of these studies, black caregivers reported less burden and less depression than white caregivers. So, in the United States at any rate, although African Americans' social network may be larger, the family's perception of social support seems somewhat problematic, and social support as measured has little explanatory value for lower perceived family burden.

Apart from this variable, Pickett, Vraniak, Cook, and Cohler (1993) attributed the finding of greater burden and depression in white families to their different level of expectation. In the research of Pickett, Vraniak, Cook, and Cohler (1993), black mothers and fathers adjusted their expectations according to their child's level of psychiatric disability, whereas white parents appeared unable to accommodate themselves to diminished expectations. "White parents may hold some abstracted normative-development expectations regarding age-appropriate behavior that may cause them to be disappointed. As a result, white parents rate their offspring's behavior as greatly delayed and in turn experience greater levels of depression and lower levels of self-worth" (p. 465).

Research and Practice Issues

Cross-cultural comparisons give rise to numerous questions. Since families continue to be the major long-term support system for persons with major mental illness, I begin with the critical issue of family interactions exemplified in the EE research.

The research on the predictive value of EE continues at a fairly steady rate, but at least two areas need considerably more study. One is the concept of low EE and whether it represents warm, accepting tolerance, as Leff and Vaughn (1985) suggest, or the potential for detached indifference (Hatfield, Spaniol, and Zipple, 1987). The emotional substrates of high EE continue to be a fertile field for exploration, particularly with the new attribution studies. Research on EE in China showed that the relationship of the respondent to the patient as parent, spouse, sibling, or child may be an independent determinant of their emotional interaction. The researchers found that among families showing high EE—as usual, a minority (33 percent) in a non-Western culture—spouses tended to show hostile criticism, whereas parents tended to be emotionally overinvolved (Phillips and Xiong, 1995). More research is clearly needed on specific role relationships of caregivers and on whether the caregiving roles of parents, spouses, siblings, and adult children are likely to vary quantitatively across cultures and to have different effects on relapse and prognosis.

To what extent is individualistic thinking implicated in high EE? Guarnaccia and Parra (1996) reported that European American families were more likely than Hispanic families to report that their family member's problem stemmed from negative personality traits—a high-EE response. This was congruent with Jenkins and Karno's findings (1992) of higher EE in Anglo families versus Hispanic families in the same city as well as similar comparison populations (Lefley, 1992). As Hooley (1987) and Barrowclough, Johnston, and Tarrier (1994) have noted, the high EE so normative in Western cultures appears to reflect familial attributions by which mentally ill persons are perceived as being in control of and capable of changing their symptomatic behaviors. White American families seem to be more disposed toward individualistic thinking, which presumes freedom of choice and personal responsibility (Miller, 1994). In this respect, white American families seem more likely than ethnic minority families to be critical of their relative's failures (Jenkins and Karno, 1992) and more disappointed in their aspirations (Pickett, Vraniak, Cook, and Cohler, 1993).

Questions remain about interactive variables. For example, are studies based on racial and ethnic diversity doing enough to control for social class or socioeconomic status (SES)? Biegel, Milligan, and Putnam (1991) found no differences in home caregiving by race when they carefully controlled for SES. Pruchno, Patrick, and Burant (1997) found that SES, rather than race, was the critical variable in caregiver burden and caregiver satisfaction. The relationship of SES to normative expectations, and of expectations to perceived burden, are clearly areas that require further exploration. Are all of these variables nested in culture, or do they disappear when social class is carefully controlled?

Are there universals in caregiver burden that transcend ethnicity? Almost all studies have found that the patient's level of behavioral problems was a significant predictor of caregiver burden for both black and white respondents. In the study by Biegel, Milligan, and Putnam (1991), the most frequently reported items by both black and white caregivers related to clients' dependency, caregiver strain (overall worry, together with lack of appreciation from patients), and family disruption due to the stress of multiple roles and responsibilities. Guarnaccia and Parra (1996) similarly found that families' dissatisfaction with the service delivery system was the same for all ethnic groups: "Many families, in discussing their experience with hospitalizing their family members, reported deep frustrations with the processes of commitment. Their own experience with and assessment of their family member was discounted by hospital staff and admission refused in spite of the families' feeling that significant deterioration has occurred. . . . The frustration many families expressed about getting family members help in a crisis was palpable during the interview" (p. 253).

Uniform complaints about services that transcend ethnic boundaries clearly call for remediation. But the other sources of data examined in this sourcebook require considerable thought, both in terms of interpretation and in applications, including deciding on appropriate responses. Different normative expectations, differences in perceived burden and reported distress—some of which may be related to SES rather than ethnicity—are issues that necessitate further exploration. What do these differences mean for discharge planning, for caregiving, and for mental health policy planning? What are the implications of these findings for clinical interventions? If individualistic thinking is related to a presumption of the patient's control and accountability and manifested in high-EE behavior, how can this be dealt with in practice?

Psychoeducational interventions have of course targeted reduction of high EE in relatives who manifest this behavior, but so far we have done very little in the way of educating families in how to cope practically and emotionally with the demands of mental illness. Psychoeducational interventions, despite their documented success in deterring relapse (Dixon and Lehman, 1995), were developed largely as part of research projects, and there is little evidence that they have been translated into standard clinical practice. Psychoeducational approaches can be culturally adapted and are demonstrably useful for ethnic minority groups in the United States. Jordan, Lewellen, and Vandiver

(1995) have discussed special considerations when working with African American, Mexican American, and Laotian families. Rivera (1988) has discussed adaptations to Hispanic culture, and Fowler (1992) has discussed adaptations to Caribbean cultures. Both Rivera and Fowler have added social activities to their psychoeducational meetings, thus expanding the social networks within their culturally homogeneous groups. Despite the overwhelmingly white composition of family support groups, a Pennsylvania study of support groups for families of persons with mental illness found that educated nonwhite women were more likely than less educated white women to be attracted to joining such groups (Mannion, Meisel, Solomon, and Draine, 1996).

Psychoeducational interventions and family education have well-developed technologies that, with appropriate adaptations, seem to be transferable across ethnicities and across cultures as well (Dixon and Lehman, 1995). All the models have common components, including educating the family about the illness, offering supportive understanding of the family experience, teaching behavior management techniques, and discussing problem-solving strategies. Although the operative variables in the success of family interventions have not been thoroughly explored, it does seem that no matter one's culture, knowing something about a family member's illness gives one a greater sense of competence in managing it. Presumably such understanding also reduces levels of anxiety and desperation, generating a calmer ambience for both family and patient.

It remains crucial that mental health facilities offer family education and support groups, or referrals to these resources, to all families of their patients. The research suggests that hospital admission policies and staff attitudes seem to be universal sources of frustration that require attention and remediation. Regardless of cultural differences between minority and white families in terms of internal versus external locus of control (and with American minority groups we do not know to what extent such cognitions have been imposed not by culture but by historical oppression), most minority families want some say over the events that shape their lives. The best way to do this is through membership in advocacy organizations such as the National Alliance for the Mentally Ill (NAMI) or the mental health associations. NAMI continues to expand its outreach efforts to ethnic minority groups, attracting affiliates and support groups for culturally specific memberships. The well-being of persons with mental illness and their families, however, rests on knowledge that is universal and on advocacy and initiatives that are inclusive of all cultural groups.

References

Barrowclough, C., Johnston, M., and Tarrier, N. "Attributions, Expressed Emotion, and Patient Relapse: An Attributional Model of Relatives' Response to Schizophrenic Illness." *Behavior Therapy,* 1994, 25, 67–88.
Barrowclough, C., Johnston, M., and Tarrier, N. "Distress, Expressed Emotion, and Attributions of Relatives of Schizophrenic Patients." Unpublished paper, Department of Clinical Psychology, School of Psychiatry, University of Manchester, England, 1995.

Biegel, D. E., Milligan, S., and Putnam, P. "The Role of Race in Family Caregiving of Persons with Mental Illness: Predictors of Caregiver Burden." In National Association of State Mental Health Program Directors, NASMHPD Research Institute, Inc., *Second Annual Conference on State Mental Health Agency Services Research, October 2–4, 1991.* Arlington, Va.: National Association of State Mental Health Program Directors, 1991.

Brewin, C. R. "Changes in Attribution and Expressed Emotion Among the Relatives of Patients with Schizophrenia." *Psychological Medicine,* 1994, *24,* 905–911.

Dixon, L. B., and Lehman, A. F. "Family Interventions for Schizophrenia." *Schizophrenia Bulletin,* 1995, *21,* 631–643.

Fowler, L. "Family Psychoeducation: Chronic Psychiatrically Ill Caribbean Patients." *Journal of Psychosocial Nursing,* 1992, *30,* 27–32.

Guarnaccia, P. J., and Parra, P. "Ethnicity, Social Status, and Families' Experiences of Caring for a Mentally Ill Family Member." *Community Mental Health Journal,* 1996, *32* (2), 243–260.

Hatfield, A. B., Spaniol, L., and Zipple, A. M. "Expressed Emotion: A Family Perspective." *Schizophrenia Bulletin,* 1987, *13,* 221–226.

Hooley, J. M. "The Nature and Origins of Expressed Emotion." In K. Hahlweg and M. J. Goldstein (eds.), *Understanding Mental Disorders: The Contribution of Family Interaction Research.* New York: Family Process, 1987.

Horwitz, A. V., and Reinhard, S. C. "Ethnic Differences in Caregiving Duties and Burdens Among Parents and Siblings of Persons with Severe Mental Illnesses." *Journal of Health and Social Behavior,* 1995, *36,* 138–150.

Iwamasa, G. Y. "Asian Americans." In S. Friedman (ed.), *Cultural Issues in the Treatment of Anxiety.* New York: Guilford Press, 1997.

Jenkins, J. H., and Karno, M. "The Meaning of Expressed Emotion: Theoretical Issues Raised by Cross-Cultural Research." *American Journal of Psychiatry,* 1992, *149,* 9–21.

Jordan, C., Lewellen, A., and Vandiver, V. "Psychoeducation for Minority Families: A Social Work Perspective." *International Journal of Mental Health,* 1995, *23* (4), 27–43.

Leff, J. *Psychiatry Around the Globe.* (2nd ed.) London: Gaskell, 1988.

Leff, J., and Vaughn, C. *Expressed Emotion in Families.* New York: Guilford Press, 1985.

Lefley, H. P. "Expressed Emotion: Conceptual, Clinical, and Social Policy Issues." *Hospital and Community Psychiatry,* 1992, *43,* 591–598.

Lefley, H. P. *Family Caregiving in Mental Illness.* Thousand Oaks, Calif.: Sage, 1996.

Mannion, E., Meisel, M., Solomon, P., and Draine, J. "A Comparative Analysis of Families with Mentally Ill Relatives: Support Group Members Versus Non-Members." *Psychiatric Rehabilitation Journal,* 1996, *20,* 43–50.

Martyns-Yellowe, I. S. "The Burden of Schizophrenia on the Family: A Study from Nigeria." *British Journal of Psychiatry,* 1992, *161,* 779–782.

Miller, J. G. "Cultural Diversity in the Morality of Caring: Individually Oriented Versus Duty-Based Interpersonal Moral Codes." *Cross-Cultural Research,* 1994, *28* (1), 3–39.

Milstein, G., Guarnaccia, P., and Midlarsky, E. "Ethnic Differences in the Interpretation of Mental Illness: Perspectives of Caregivers." In J. R. Greenley (ed.), *The Family and Mental Illness.* Research in Community and Mental Health, no. 8. Greenwich, Conn.: JAI Press, 1995.

Phillips, M. R., and Xiong, W. "Expressed Emotion in Mainland China: Chinese Families with Schizophrenic Patients." *International Journal of Mental Health,* 1995, *24* (3), 54–75.

Pickett, S. A., Vraniak, D. A., Cook, J. A., and Cohler, B. A. "Strength in Adversity: Blacks Bear Burden Better Than Whites." *Professional Psychology: Research and Practice,* 1993, *24,* 460–467.

Pruchno, R., Patrick, J. H., and Burant, C. J. "African-American and White Mothers of Adults with Chronic Disabilities: Caregiving Burden and Satisfaction." *Family Relations,* 1997.

Rivera, C. "Culturally Sensitive Aftercare Services for Chronically Mentally Ill Hispanics: The Case of the Psychoeducation Treatment Model." *Hispanic Research Center Research Bulletin,* 1988, *11* (1), 1–9.

Shankar, R., and Menon, M. S. "Interventions with Families of People with Schizophrenia: The Issues Facing a Community Rehabilitation Center in India." *Psychosocial Rehabilitation Journal*, 1991, *15*, 85–90.

Steuve, A., Vine, P., and Streuning, E. "Perceived Burden Among Caregivers of Adults with Serious Mental Illness: Comparison of Black, Hispanic, and White Families." *American Journal of Orthopsychiatry*, 1997, *67*, 199–209.

Streit, U. "Nathan's Ethnopsychoanalytic Therapy: Characteristics, Discoveries, and Challenges to Western Psychotherapy." *Transcultural Psychiatry*, 1997, *34*, 321–343.

Triandis, H. *Individualism and Collectivism*. Boulder, Colo.: Westview Press, 1995.

Westermeyer, J., and Janca, A. "Language, Culture and Psychopathology: Conceptual and Methodological Issues." *Transcultural Psychiatry*, 1997, *34*, 291–311.

HARRIET P. LEFLEY is professor of psychiatry and behavioral sciences, University of Miami School of Medicine.

Name Index

SUBJECT INDEX

Access, to mental health services, 57, 64. *See also* by specific ethnic group
Administrative staff culture, 22
Administrators: collaboration training of, 28; values about families of, 22
Adult children, mentally ill, 11–12
Advocacy/support groups: Caucasian membership of, 63, 69; community organizations and, 70–71; cultural competence and, 69–71; friendships in, 68–69; member evolution in, 13; minorities in, 63–65; operation of, 9; origins of, 6–7; outreach by, 104; satisfaction with, 69; women members in, 104. See also Support groups, minority families and (study)
African American families: accommodation of illness by, 11; burdens on, 51–52, 101; caregiver age in, 47; caregiving ideology of, 64; community outreach programs for, 70–71; conceptualization of illness of, 52–54; day programs and, 101; income level of, 49; interventions for, 10; pathways to care of, 54–55; patient living arrangements in, 49, 101; support networks of, 50–51, 59, 68; unmet service needs of, 64
Alcohol/drug abuse: mental illness and, 90–91; Native Americans and, 90–92
Alliance for the Mentally Ill (AMI), 34, 49
American Indian families. *See* Native American families
American Psychiatric Association, 21
Asian American families: access to services of, 64; caregiving ideology of, 64;
Assertive community treatment (ACT), 10
Asylums, 5–6
Autonomy/independence, multicultural patterns in, 55, 70

Bias, 11–12. *See also* Stigma
Bilateral training approach: administrators and, 28; barriers to collaboration and, 26–28; brainstorming and, 28; cofacilitation in, 27; collaborative basis for, 25; family factors and, 26; joint groups in, 26–27; mutual empathy and, 26; peer learning and, 26; restructuring attitudes in, 25–26; role modeling/reversal and, 26; role-playing and, 28; scheduling problems and, 26–27
Biopsychosocial explanatory models, 6
Bipolar disorder, 90–92
British families, expressed emotion and, 98–99
Buffalo Psychiatric Hospital, New York, 25
Burden, family: assessment of, 56; expectation and, 101–102; expressed emotion and, 100; financial, 52; minority families and, 51–52, 101; support networks and, 101; trauma as, 36

Caregivers: aging, 47; carers and, 97; female, 48
Caregiving: increased role of, 55; minority families' view of, 64
Caregiving, multicultural aspects of (study): caregiver age and, 47; family income and, 49; family profile, 47–49; family social characteristics and, 47–49; feminization of, 48; financial burden and, 51–52; illness conceptualization and, 52–54; implications of, 55–59; other burdens and, 52; pathways to care and, 54–55; patient social characteristics and, 49–50; social support networks and, 50–51
Carers, 97
Case management: family interventions and, 9–10; service needs of, 69
Caucasians: mental health ideology of, 63–64; support group participation of, 63, 65, 69. *See also* European American families
Center for Mental Health Services (CMHS), 90, 92
Clinical practice. *See* Families, working with
Clinicians. *See* Mental health practitioners
Collaboration, family-provider, 17–18, 20–22, 25–28. *See also* Bilateral training approach
Collectivist culture, 98. *See also* Sociocentric culture
Communication: family-professional, 81–82; nonverbal versus verbal, 79; strategies in helping process, 85

and, 21–22; shift in view of, 7; socio-centric versus individualistic, 98–99; stereotypes of, 38–39; trauma model of recovery and, 36; white versus minority, 11, 45–46. *See also* Burden, family; Families, working with; Family-provider relationship; Interventions, family; *and by specific ethnic group*
Family-Aided Assertive Community Treatment (FACT), 10
Family advocacy/support groups. *See* Advocacy/support groups
Family caregiver movement, 34
Family caregiving. *See* Caregiving
Family consultation, 8
Family culture: ethnicity and, 10; family interventions and, 10–11. *See also* Culture; *and by specific ethnic group*
Family education, 8–9, 33–34, 36, 58–59, 104. *See also* NAMI Family-to-Family Education Program
Family-provider relationships: administrative culture and, 22; challenges in, 28–29; collaboration in, 17–18, 25–29; cultural components of, 18; experienced families and, 24–25; family behavior and, 23–25; family beliefs and, 23–25; family values and, 22–24; financial aspects of, 22; new families and, 22–24. *See also* Bilateral training approach; Family(ies); Service providers
Family systems theory, 6
Family therapy: bias in, 12; immigrant groups and, 10; origins of, 6
Financial planning programs, 9
Framing event, 23

Healing: of trauma, 37, 40; traditional cultures and, 98–99
Help seeking: cultural differences in, 46–47; cultural perceptions of illness and, 79–80; family values and, 22–23; pathways to, 46, 54–55
Hispanic American families: access to services of, 64; burdens on, 51–52; caregiver age in, 47; conceptualization of illness of, 52–54, 64, 100; income level of, 49; interdependence in, 70; pathways to care of, 54; patient living arrangements in, 49; psychoeducation for, 58; religion/spiritualism of, 64; residential programs and, 101; support

networks of, 50–51, 59. *See also* Mexican American families
Homogenization, theory of, 65

Immigrant groups, 10
Independence. *See* Autonomy/independence
Individualistic culture, 98, 102
Indochinese: Cambodians, 76; culture of, 76–77; demographics/immigration of, 75; health/wellness beliefs of, 80; Laotians, 76; mental disorders among, 77–79; nonverbal communication of, 79; religion/spiritualism and, 76, 80; secretiveness of, 80; studies on, 75; traditional healing methods of, 80–81; Vietnamese, 76–77
Indochinese families: assimilation process of, 86; clinician response to, 75; coping strategies for, 84–85; delayed treatment and, 79; family structure of, 77, 79; interventions for, 83; long-term support for, 84; programs for, 86; psychoeducation for, 83–84; service underutilization by, 80; support networks of, 77, 80–81; view of mental illness of, 78, 80, 82. *See also* Indochinese families, working with
Indochinese families, working with: assessing clients/families, 82–83; choosing interventions, 83; culturally relevant approach with, 81–86; enhancing clinician-family communication, 81–82; family expectations and, 82; family roles/structure and, 79; health/illness beliefs and, 79–80, 82; help-seeking attempts and, 82; nonconfrontational-directive approach with, 85–86; nonverbal communication and, 79; offering coping strategies, 84–85; primary themes in, 85–86; providing psychoeducation/support, 83–84; traditional support systems and, 80–81; using communication strategies, 85
Interconnectedness/involvement, multicultural patterns in, 56
Interventions, family: advocacy/support groups, 9, 13; assertive community treatment and, 10; availability/accessibility of, 12; case management services and, 9–10; culture of, 12–13; defining, 7; degree of alliance and, 12; design/use of, 12–13; ethnicity and, 10; family consultation, 8; family culture and,

traditional economy of, 94–95; treatment referrals for, 92; tribal differences and, 89
Native American Family Project, 90, 92–93
Negativity, provider, 11–12, 20–21
Networks. *See* Advocacy/support groups; - Support networks
New psychiatry, 35
Nonverbal communication, cultural factors in, 79

Patients: expressed emotion and, 6, 93, 100; family therapy and, 6; as loved ones, 97–98; minority families view of, 11, 45; separation from family of, 5–6, 10
Peer learning, 26
Post-traumatic stress disorder, 78
Primary intervention, 36
Privatization, of mental health care, 91
Psychiatric illness. *See* Mental illness
Psychic healing, 37, 40
Psychodynamic paradigm, 97
Psychodynamic theory, 6
Psychoeducation, 7–8, 33, 36, 58, 83–84, 103–104. *See also by specific ethnic group*
Psychosocial interventions, 6. *See also* Interventions, family

Remission, of mental illness, 94–95
Respite care, 52
Role modeling, 26
Role reversal, 26
Role-playing, 28

Schizophrenia: expressed emotion and, 93, 100; family conception of illness as, 52; among Indochinese, 78; lifetime course of, 92; medical model of, 58–59; Native American populations and, 90, 92–93; treatment guidelines for, 92; WHO study of, 92–93
Secondary intervention, 35–36
Separation, patient-family, 5–6, 10
Service providers: administrative staff culture and, 22; attitudes toward families of, 20–21; behavioral norms of, 21–22; beliefs about profession of, 21; family behavior and, 23–24; family beliefs

about, 23; job values of, 19–20. *See also* Family-provider relationships; Mental health professionals; Professional culture
Service providers. *See* Mental health professionals
Siblings, interventions for, 11
Sociocentric culture, 98
Spouses, interventions for, 11
Stereotypes, of mental health, 38–39. *See also* Stigma
Stigma: advocacy campaigns against, 13; clinician-patient barrier and, 75; families and, 7, 14. *See also* Bias; Stereotypes
Supplemental Security Income (SSI), 94
Support groups, minority families and (study): analysis/results, 67–68; community outreach programs and, 70–71; cultural competence issues and, 69–71; discussion, 68–69; friendship development and, 68–69; information needs and, 69; limitations, 68; measures, 67; method, 65–68; satisfaction with, 69; subjects, 65–67
Support networks: assessment of, 56; cross-ethnic studies and, 100–101; European American family, 49–51, 59; families as, 99; family burden and, 101; family perception of, 101; help seeking and, 101; of Indochinese families, 77, 80–81; mental illness and, 99; minority family, 49–51, 59, 64, 101; supportive resources and, 101. *See also* Advocacy/support groups
Supportive family counseling, 8

Traditional culture. *See* Sociocentric culture
Training, clinical, 19–20. *See also* Bilateral training approach
Training and Education Center (TEC), 8
Trauma: family burden of, 36; healing of, 37, 40
Trauma model of recovery: families and, 36; NAMI Family-to-Family Education Program and, 36–37; psychic healing and, 37; secondary intervention framework of, 35
Vocational training programs, 57–58

World Health Organization (WHO), 92

ORDERING INFORMATION

NEW DIRECTIONS FOR MENTAL HEALTH SERVICES is a series of paperback books that presents timely and readable volumes on subjects of concern to clinicians, administrators, and others involved in the care of the mentally disabled. Each volume is devoted to one topic and includes a broad range of authoritative articles written by noted specialists in the field. Books in the series are published quarterly in Spring, Summer, Fall, and Winter and are available for purchase by subscription and individually.

SUBSCRIPTIONS cost $63.00 for individuals (a savings of 37 percent over single-copy prices) and $105.00 for institutions, agencies, and libraries. Standing orders are accepted. New York residents, add local sales tax for subscriptions. (For subscriptions outside the United States, add $7.00 for shipping via surface mail or $25.00 for air mail. Orders *must be prepaid* in U.S. dollars by check drawn on a U.S. bank or charged to VISA, MasterCard, or American Express.)

SINGLE COPIES cost $25.00 plus shipping (see below) when payment accompanies order. California, New Jersey, New York, and Washington, D.C., residents, please include appropriate sales tax. Canadian residents, add GST and any local taxes. Billed orders will be charged shipping and handling. No billed shipments to post office boxes. (Orders from outside the United States *must be prepaid* in U.S. dollars by check drawn on a U.S. bank or charged to VISA, MasterCard, or American Express.)

SHIPPING (SINGLE COPIES ONLY): $30.00 and under, add $5.50; to $50.00, add $6.50; to $75.00, add $7.50; to $100.00, add $9.00; to $150.00, add $10.00.

ALL PRICES are subject to change.

DISCOUNTS FOR QUANTITY ORDERS are available. Please write to the address below for information.

ALL ORDERS must include either the name of an individual or an official purchase order number. Please submit your order as follows:
Subscriptions: specify series and year subscription is to begin
Single copies: include individual title code (such as MHS59)

MAIL ALL ORDERS TO:
Jossey-Bass Publishers
350 Sansome Street
San Francisco, California 94104–1342

FOR SUBSCRIPTION SALES OUTSIDE OF THE UNITED STATES, contact any international subscription agency or Jossey-Bass directly.

OTHER TITLES AVAILABLE IN THE
NEW DIRECTIONS FOR MENTAL HEALTH SERVICES SERIES
H. Richard Lamb, Editor-in-Chief